Inside
Chiropractic

Consumer Health Library®
Series Editor: Stephen Barrett, M.D.
Technical Editor: Manfred Kroger, Ph.D.

Other titles in this series:

Inside
Chiropractic

A Patient's Guide

SAMUEL HOMOLA, D.C.
Edited by STEPHEN BARRETT, M.D.

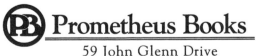

Prometheus Books
59 John Glenn Drive
Amherst, New York 14228-2197

Published 1999 by Prometheus Books

03 02 01 00 99   5 4 3 2 1

Library of Congress Cataloging-in-Publication Data

Homola, Samuel.
    Inside chiropractic : a patient's guide / Samuel Homola ; edited by Stephen
Barrett.
        p.   cm.
    Includes bibliographical references and index.
    ISBN 1–57392–698–1 (alk. paper)
    1. Chiropractic—Evaluation. 2. Medical misconceptions. 3. Consumer
education. I. Barrett, Stephen, 1933–   . II. Title.
RZ242.H65   1999
615.5'34—dc21   99–19397
                                                                        CIP

Printed in the United States of America on acid-free paper

Contents

Preface

Chiropractic, which celebrated its centennial in 1995, is a curious mixture of science and pseudoscience, sense and nonsense. Much of it is based on the theory that misaligned spinal bones produce nerve interference that causes disease. Many chiropractors claim that correcting these misalignments ("subluxations") can restore health and that regular spinal adjustments are essential to maintain it.

Neither logic nor scientific evidence supports such a belief. Although spinal manipulation can relieve certain types of back pain, neck pain, and other musculoskeletal symptoms, there is no scientific evidence that it can restore or maintain general health. As a result of expressing my opinions on this subject, I have been called a chiropractic heretic.

The chiropractic profession has little tolerance for dissension. Its nonsense remains unchallenged by its leaders and has not been denounced in its journals. In fact, many chiropractic journals continue to publish articles that attempt to justify subluxation theory. Although progress has been made, the profession still has one foot lightly planted in science and the other firmly rooted in cultism. Without appropriate criticism, the good in chiropractic will never be sifted out, and competent chiropractors will not receive the recognition they deserve.

This book denounces the cultism in chiropractic but supports the appropriate use of spinal manipulation and the research efforts required to solidify its scientific basis. If you are contemplating or receiving chiropractic care, *Inside Chiropractic* might help you protect both your pocketbook and your health.

Samuel Homola, D.C.

Acknowledgments

This book is dedicated to my wife, Martha, who stood by me all these years. The following people provided valuable help:

Project managers	Christine Kramer, Mary A. Read
	Prometheus Books
Legal advisor	Michael Botts, Esq., Ames, Iowa
Technical editor	Manfred Kroger, Ph.D.,
	Professor of Food Science
	The Pennsylvania State University
Consultants	Charles E. DuVall, Jr., D.C., Board Chairman
	National Council Against Health Fraud
	William T. Jarvis, Ph.D., Professor of
	Health Promotion and Education
	Loma Linda University
	Ronald L. Slaughter, D.C., Co-Founder
	National Association for Chiropractic Medicine
Line drawings	Bibiana Neal, Panama City, Florida
Photographs	Tom Needham, Panama City, Florida

I also thank the many others who shared their experiences and contributed documents and other information important to this project.

A Note about References

Throughout this work, the numbers within brackets [ ] refer to references listed in Appendix E. The first page of a cited passage from a book may be indicated by a number after a colon, e.g., [23:57].

About the Author

Samuel Homola, D.C., has been a practicing chiropractor for forty-three years. He is the author of eleven other books, including *Bonesetting, Chiropractic, and Cultism*; *Backache: Home Treatment and Prevention*; and *Muscle Training for Athletes*. He has also written many articles for magazines and journals, ranging from *Cosmopolitan* and *Scholastic Coach* to *Chiropractic Technique* and *Archives of Family Medicine*. Now retired, he lives in Panama City, Florida, with his wife, Martha.

About the Editor

Stephen Barrett, M.D., a retired psychiatrist who resides in Allentown, Pennsylvania, is a nationally renowned author, editor, and consumer advocate. He has been collecting information about chiropractic for more than thirty years. He is board chairman of Quackwatch, Inc., a board member of the National Council Against Health Fraud, and chairman of the council's Task Force on Victim Redress. His forty-six books include *The Health Robbers: A Close Look at Quackery in America*; *The Vitamin Pushers: How the "Health Food" Industry Is Selling America a Bill of Goods*; *Reader's Guide to "Alternative" Health Methods*; and five editions of the college textbook *Consumer Health: A Guide to Intelligent Decisions*. He operates three Web sites: Quackwatch (http://www.quackwatch.com), Chirobase (http://www.chirobase.org), and MLM Watch (http://www.mlmwatch.org). He can be reached at (610) 437-1795.

Important Definitions

- **Vertebra.** Bony segment of the spine that encircles and helps protect the spinal cord and nerves. The plural of vertebra is vertebrae.
- **Cervical vertebrae.** The seven bones in the neck area of the spine.
- **Thoracic vertebrae.** The twelve bones in the upper-back portion of the spine.
- **Lumbar vertebrae.** The five bones in the lower-back portion of the spine.
- **Sacrum.** The triangular bone that serves as a base for the spinal column and connects the pelvic bones.
- **Subluxation.** Medical term for partial dislocation of a bone. Chiropractors define "vertebral subluxation" in many ways. Throughout this book—unless otherwise noted—the word "subluxation" refers to the chiropractic concept of vertebral subluxation.
- **Manipulation.** Manual manipulation to loosen or mobilize vertebrae. Many chiropractors who purport to correct subluxations to improve health prefer to describe their treatment as "spinal adjustments."
- **Palmerian.** Pertaining to the ideas and practices of chiropractic's founder (D.D. Palmer) and developer (his son B.J. Palmer).
- **Straight chiropractors ("straights").** Chiropractors who cling to Palmerian doctrines that most health problems are caused by misaligned spinal bones ("vertebral subluxations") and are correctable by manual manipulation of the spine.
- **Mixer chiropractors ("mixers").** Chiropractors who use physical therapy and other nondrug treatment methods in addition to manual manipulation of the spine.
- **American Chiropractic Association (ACA).** The largest chiropractic association, representing "mixer" chiropractors.
- **International Chiropractors Association (ICA).** The second-largest chiropractic association, representing "straight" chiropractors.

1

My Personal Story

I have practiced chiropractic full-time for forty-three years. Throughout my career, the only conditions I treated were mechanical-type back and neck pain and other musculoskeletal problems. My work has been appreciated by my patients and, in recent years, by many physicians. But most chiropractors familiar with my writings consider me a heretic because I openly criticize chiropractic dogma.

My father, Joseph Homola, was also a chiropractor. He came to America from Czechoslovakia at about the age of eighteen, entered the Palmer School of Chiropractic at the age of thirty-two, and graduated in 1920 after an eighteen-month course of instruction. My earliest recollection of his work is his arrest for practicing chiropractic in Dothan, Alabama. I was only five years old at that time, but I recall waiting anxiously for his return home late that night.

Before chiropractic licensing laws were passed, thousands of chiropractors were prosecuted for practicing medicine without a license. The typical penalty was a small fine, but many were briefly jailed. Fortunately, my father was treating a member of the judge's family, so no charges were filed and my father was able to continue in practice, even though Alabama did not enact a chiropractic licensing law during his lifetime.

Chiropractic is based on beliefs that spinal problems are the underlying cause of disease. Its founder, Daniel David Palmer, had declared in 1895 that the basic cause of ill health was nerve interference caused by displaced vertebrae, and that the basic remedy was spinal adjustment. He rejected the germ theory and had an aversion to drugs, surgery, and medical diagnosis.

The school my father attended had been founded by D.D. Palmer and developed by his son Bartlett Joshua ("B.J."). Like virtually all of its graduates, my father treated the gamut of human ailments with spinal adjustments. His office was located above a movie theater in downtown Dothan. A small sign that said "J. Homola, Chiropractor" hung over the doorway at sidewalk level.

In those days, chiropractic was represented as a "new science" that treated disease by correcting misaligned vertebrae that were pinching spinal nerves. Many people thought of chiropractors as quacks, and this perception was reinforced by the medical community. Nevertheless, chiropractic's theory appealed to many, especially those who had diseases unhealed by medical practice. Few people knew enough to judge chiropractors one way or the other.

Early Observations

Most of my father's patients were chronically ill. Many had back pain or a stiff neck. On Saturdays, when the farmers came to town, my father always had a few new patients who had heard by word-of-mouth that chiropractic adjustments could cure just about anything. It seemed logical to these hard-working folks that when painful "locking" of the back occurred, a chiropractor who could pop the spine could solve the problem. And my father thought so, too. He often told me that while growing up in the Bohemian district of Czechoslovakia, he regularly walked barefoot up and down his father's back to relieve the aches and pains of farming.

Many of my father's patients experienced sudden and dramatic relief of back pain after their treatment. Many others who recovered from self-limiting illnesses also attributed their recovery to his adjustments, believing that pinched nerves had been relieved. As his office practice grew and his reputation spread, my father received requests for house calls, often from out of town, and even from out of state. During my grammar school years, I often accompanied him on weekends when he drove through Georgia or Alabama to treat homebound or bedridden patients, most of whom suffered from chronic conditions such as weakness or paralysis from a stroke.

My father's office equipment consisted of a chiropractic treatment table and a combination ultraviolet and heat lamp. For house calls, he would bring a folding table that separated into two pieces. The table would be set up in the bedroom or living room with a chair turned on its side, covered with pillows, and placed between the two sections. This setup permitted some downward movement of the spine when my father pressed on the lower back to treat back pain.

My job was to find a suitable chair and set up the tables. Then, with the patient lying facedown, my father would quickly pop the patient's neck and upper back. After that, we often would stay for lunch or dinner, which was a real treat because farmers usually served fresh ham or fried chicken and homegrown vegetables. Many of the farmers who came to town for treatment would pay my father with eggs, live chickens, cane syrup, and other staples from the farm. We were particularly well supplied with cane syrup.

My father believed that his methods were highly effective. Yet, as time passed, he developed doubts about chiropractic's basic theory. He once told me that "You couldn't get a vertebra out of place with a crowbar." When any of us were sick, however, he always gave us a chiropractic adjustment, which usually consisted of popping our neck and upper back. But sometimes he used medical doctors. When his four children were born, he called for medical assistance. And when I developed pneumonia as a small child, he called in a medical doctor. Fortunately, I survived the infection despite the fact that antibiotics were not yet available.

For the most part, however, my father was influenced by B.J. Palmer's teachings. My family was not permitted to use drugs or get shots. My father believed that the body would heal itself and that chiropractic adjustments would help prevent disease. When we got sick, we simply stayed home and got daily chiropractic adjustments. When my younger brother Bill was five or six years old, he fell from a porch and landed on his head, causing severe neck pain that prevented him from moving his head. My parents nursed him at home until he recovered. The seriousness of Bill's injury did not become apparent until many years later when I x-rayed his neck in my office. A deformity involving the top two vertebrae in his neck indicated that they had been fractured and that Bill was very fortunate to have made a full recovery. I'm sure that my father, who did not have an x-ray machine, was unaware that Bill's neck had been broken.

My recovery from pneumonia and my brother's recovery from a broken neck had nothing to do with chiropractic treatment. Such recoveries are a tribute to the remarkable healing power of the body. Of course, today, with all that medical science has to offer for treating serious illness or injury, it would be senseless to reject proper medical care.

Entering Chiropractic School

As the years passed, my father's doubts about chiropractic grew. When I was in high school and thinking about a career, he sometimes advised me not to follow in his footsteps. After serving in the Navy for four years during the Korean War, I was eligible to attend college under the G.I. Bill. I considered other health-related fields but was drawn more strongly to chiropractic. I felt that my knowledge of chiropractic and my interest in health-related matters would serve me well. I rationalized that much of the criticism of chiropractic was medically instigated and not entirely accurate or deserved. Surely chiropractic had changed for the better, since the course of study was now four years and chiropractors had achieved licensure in forty-three states.

My first two years at Lincoln Chiropractic College included courses in anatomy, biochemistry, physiology, pathology, and other basic sciences. These subjects are vital for medical students, because they provide the foundation for understanding many diseases and their treatment, especially drug treatment. But most had little relevance to chiropractic practice. After all, if all health problems emanate from spinal problems and can be fixed by spinal adjustment, what happens at the cellular level is unimportant.

My Doubts Begin

At the start of my second year at Lincoln, I began to have serious doubts and to worry about my future. As I learned more about chiropractic "philosophy," I started to suspect that chiropractic's basic theory might be wrong and that my father's doubts were well founded. The school taught that spinal adjustments were the only treatment needed. Physical therapy was not taught and was thought to have little value because "it relieves symptoms rather than correcting the cause of disease." We were taught to adjust the vertebrae to remove nerve interference so that the body could heal itself, regardless of what disease the patient might have. Today, this is still known as "The Big Idea." One day, a Lincoln student suffered an epileptic seizure during class and fell to the floor. The instructor, who happened to be the school's president, walked over, popped the poor fellow's neck, and left him convulsing on the floor. My doubts multiplied.

I had decided to practice in Florida, which required passage of a basic sciences examination before taking the chiropractic state board exams. (This requirement no longer exists.) Chiropractic students normally waited until the end of their final year to take the exam, but passing it sooner would enable me to concentrate on orthopedics and physical therapy. So I studied hard, often reading far ahead of class lessons. At the end of my first two years at Lincoln, I took the basic science test and passed it.

My Skepticism Deepens

Nothing I encountered in chiropractic school persuaded me that spinal adjustments had any effect on general health. My basic science studies increased my skepticism. One of our required textbooks was *Best & Taylor's Physiological Basis of Medical Practice,* a highly respected work used in medical schools. Although the school taught that adjusting the neck would stimulate the parasympathetic nervous system, the book stated:

> It is very questionable whether the vagus can be stimulated by pressure through the overlying tissues, for in operations upon the neck, even pinching the nerve with forceps does not stimulate it; and in animals, the vagus is relatively unresponsive to mechanical stimulation. [25]

Then I read *Pottenger's Symptoms of Visceral Disease*, which indicated that the autonomic system could function independently of the spinal cord [145]. We were being taught that all bodily functions were controlled through their connection to the spine. But the book cited animal experiments in which the autonomic nervous system (the part of the nervous system that controls nonvoluntary functions) kept working even though its connections to the spinal cord were completely severed. I also learned that tissue cells can function independently of the nervous system and depend upon chemical reactions fueled by tissue fluid nutrients.

It soon became apparent to me that the function of an organ depended upon biochemical reactions as well as nerve supply from a wide distribution of nerves that are interconnected with many other nerves and nerve centers outside the spinal column. While the nervous system coordinated functions, many functions did not require a nerve supply. Thus it seemed improbable to me that a single spinal nerve affected by a misaligned ("subluxated") vertebra could be a factor in causing internal organs to become diseased.

Chiropractic theory stated that a subluxated vertebra pinching a spinal nerve could have a harmful effect on a certain organ. Our instructors, almost all of whom were chiropractors, ignored the fact that hormonal and other biochemical factors regulated cellular functions throughout the body. We were taught the meric system—a creation of B.J. Palmer and a colleague—

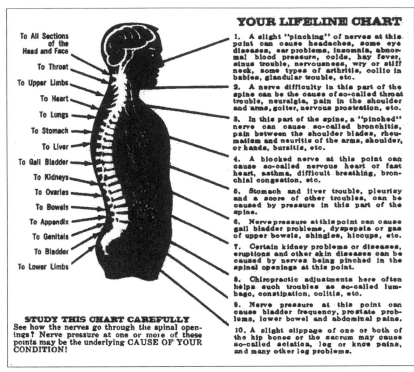

YOUR LIFELINE CHART

To All Sections of the Head and Face

To Throat

To Upper Limbs

To Heart

To Lungs

To Stomach

To Liver

To Gall Bladder

To Kidneys

To Ovaries

To Bowels

To Appendix

To Genitals

To Bladder

To Lower Limbs

1. A slight "pinching" of nerves at this point can cause headaches, some eye diseases, ear problems, insomnia, abnormal blood pressure, colds, hay fever, sinus trouble, nervousness, wry or stiff neck, some types of arthritis, collic in babies, glandular trouble, etc.

2. A nerve difficulty in this part of the spine can be the cause of so-called throat trouble, neuralgia, pain in the shoulder and arms, goiter, nervous prostration, etc.

3. In this part of the spine, a "pinched" nerve can cause so-called bronchitis, pain between the shoulder blades, rheumatism and neuritis of the arms, shoulder, or hands, bursitis, etc.

4. A blocked nerve at this point can cause so-called nervous heart or fast heart, asthma, difficult breathing, bronchial congestion, etc.

5. Stomach and liver trouble, pleurisy and a score of other troubles, can be caused by pressure in this part of the spine.

6. Nerve pressure at this point can cause gall bladder problems, dyspepsia or gas of upper bowels, shingles, hiccups, etc.

7. Certain kidney problems or diseases, eruptions and other skin diseases can be caused by nerves being pinched in the spinal openings at this point.

8. Chiropractic adjustments here often helps such troubles as so-called lumbago, constipation, colitis, etc.

9. Nerve pressure at this point can cause bladder frequency, prostate problems, lower bowel and abdominal pains.

10. A slight slippage of one or both of the hip bones or the sacrum may cause so-called sciatica, leg or knee pains, and many other leg problems.

STUDY THIS CHART CAREFULLY
See how the nerves go through the spinal openings? Nerve pressure at one or more of these points may be the underlying CAUSE OF YOUR CONDITION!

This chart from a 1964 brochure illustrates the meric system of adjusting, which was introduced in 1909. The accompanying text states (incorrectly) that "the nervous system regulates and controls all other systems of the body" and that "a misaligned spinal vertebra can cause disease in ANY PART OF THE BODY." The brochure also claims that "nerve pressure" at one or more of the points indicated by the arrows "may be the underlying CAUSE OF YOUR CONDITION!" Charts like this contributed to the skepticism I developed during my student days.

which held that each joint of the spine can influence specific body structures; that "subluxations" of specific joints cause disease in their corresponding organs; and that specific segments of the spine were adjusted to treat specific organs and diseases (see above illustration). Although my fellow students read many of the same basic science books as I did, they assumed that "subluxations" had effects not yet explained in neurology. So they continued adjusting vertebrae as a treatment for infections and other diseases.

The more I studied, the more skeptical I became. I went to a nearby medical school library and read books on orthopedics and back pain. The only books that focused on what I thought was appropriate use of spinal manipulation were written by orthopedic surgeons and physical medicine specialists—not chiropractors. James Mennell, M.D.'s books on joint manipulation were the most illuminating. Pain caused by restricted motion of a joint in the neck or back is usually localized in the area of the affected joint. Mennell pointed out that pain originating in a joint is sometimes referred to another part of the body and can mimic the symptoms of a visceral (internal organ) disorder. Thus the pain of a neck problem might be mistaken for the neck pain sometimes caused by angina pectoris—and relieving the neck pain might lead a chiropractor or patient to conclude that a heart problem had been cured. Mennell also pointed out that whereas a heart problem could refer pain into the neck, shoulder, and arm, a pinched spinal nerve would have no effect on the heart. Nor did he believe that manipulation could help any pathological condition of an internal organ [123]. In 1954, I photocopied pages from Mennell's books and distributed them to my fellow students. That was the beginning of my reputation as a chiropractic heretic.

Although I could no longer believe that disease could be caused by misaligned vertebrae, I was convinced that spinal manipulation was useful for some types of back pain as well as tension headache and other conditions related to tightness and other problems in muscles and joints. Yet very few medical doctors offered manipulation. Chiropractors and osteopaths did so, but most of them used it inappropriately.

My Proper Path Becomes Clear

During my final year at Lincoln College, much of my time was spent in the clinic where I used spinal adjustments to treat patients, most of whom were ambulatory and presented with common and often chronic and incurable conditions. I became skillful in manipulating the spine. However, we saw very few acute or seriously ill patients, so my clinical experience was extremely narrow.

The examination room was equipped with little more than a reflex hammer, tongue depressors, a scale for weighing patients, and a Cameron Heartometer. The treatment cubicle contained only an adjusting table. Every patient underwent a spinal examination, which consisted largely of palpation of the spine to detect "subluxated" vertebrae. X-ray examination was also commonly used to locate the subluxations, or what students perceived to be subluxations. The Heartometer was a mechanical device that recorded blood pressure and pulse rate on a graph. It was used along with a stethoscope and a standard blood pressure device (sphygmomanometer) to evaluate the heart as a preliminary to spinal adjustments.

In 1956, my classmates and I were given diplomas and turned loose to heal the sick using only spinal adjustments. I knew that was impossible, but I believed I could provide a valuable alternative. I would limit my practice to conditions for which manipulation, exercise, and other physical measures were appropriate. I would select my patients carefully and refer those who needed medical care. And I would do what I could to help develop and promote appropriate use of spinal manipulation. Wishing me the best, my father died in 1957, shortly after I opened my office in Panama City, Florida.

Progress, But Not Enough

Today, with increasing recognition of manipulation for treating back pain and widespread insurance coverage, increasing numbers of people are seeking chiropractic care. Our educational standards have increased to the point where all chiropractic colleges require two to four years of pre-professional training and most include instruction in physical therapy and other supportive measures. But the philosophy of the Palmers still enshrouds the profession. Many schools teach that subluxations (misalignments) are the major cause of disease; and most teach that spinal adjustments are effective in restoring and maintaining health. Neither of these assertions is true.

This persistence of chiropractic dogma poses a serious threat to patients. Whereas spinal manipulation is often the best treatment for back pain, excessive or inappropriate use can do more harm than good. This book, based mainly on my personal experience, can help you understand what chiropractors can and cannot do.

2

From Bonesetting
to "The Big Idea"

Chiropractic is based on the philosophy of Daniel David Palmer, who declared in 1895 that spinal misalignments are the primary cause of ill health. His recommended treatment—spinal "adjustment" or manipulation—remains chiropractic's hallmark. Palmer's method was actually not new. His distinctive aspect was the theory he gave to explain his alleged results.

Spinal manipulation has actually been practiced since ancient times. A Chinese Kung Fu document, for example, describes it in China as early as 2700 BCE [191].

Hippocrates (460–375 BCE), the Greek physician known as the "father of medicine," wrote extensively about spinal manipulation. His books *On Fractures*, *On Setting Joints by Leverage*, and *On the Articulations* reflected centuries of recorded knowledge. In the last of these, he explained how to differentiate between complete dislocations (luxations) and partial dislocations (subluxations):

> In a word, luxations and subluxations take place in different degrees, being sometimes greater and sometimes less . . . but when the bone has slipped, or been displaced to a less extent, it is easier to reduce such cases than the other. [77]

For treating spinal curvatures, he recommended placing the patient facedown on a bench "covered with robes, or anything else which is soft but does not yield much." With one strap under the arms and across the chest, and another around the knees and ankles, traction ("extension") could be applied to the patient from both ends of the bench. Then:

> The physician, or some person who is strong, and not uninstructed, should apply the palm of one hand to the hump, and then, having laid the other hand upon the former, he should make pressure, attending whether this force should be applied directly downward, or toward the head, or towards the hips. This method of applying force is particularly safe; and it is also safe for a person to sit upon the hump while the extension is made, and raising himself up, to let himself fall again on the patient. And there is nothing to prevent a person from placing a foot on the hump, and supporting his weight on it, and making gentle pressure; one of the men who is practiced in the palestra would be a proper person for doing this in a suitable manner. [77]

Another method, which Hippocrates considered "the most powerful of the mechanical means," required thrusting against the spine with a board. A hole in a piece of wood was aligned with the hump or other area of the spine undergoing treatment, which was padded with rags or a cushion. Then:

> When matters are thus adjusted, one person, or two if necessary, must press down on the end of the board, whilst others at the same time make extension and counter-extension along the body.... And the forces are applied in the natural way; for the pressure above forces the displaced parts into their place. [77]

Another common method was succussion on a ladder. The patient was strapped to a ladder—upright or upside down, depending upon the location of the dislocation. The ladder was then dropped from a height, so that the force of gravity, suddenly multiplied when the end of the ladder hit the ground, would reduce the dislocation by stretching the spine. "I could tell of other modes of succussion," Hippocrates wrote, "but I have no great confidence in them, and therefore I do not describe them."

Through the Centuries

Ambroise Parè, a sixteenth-century French surgeon, commented on Hippocrates' methods and advised his colleagues: "I do not teach any such way of giving the strappado to men, but I show the surgeon in my works, the method of reducing them safely and without great pain" [70].

One of the earliest known English works on bonesetting, *The Compleat Bone-Setter*, was written by Friar Moulton, a member of the religious order of St. Augustine. The book, revised by Robert Turner in 1656, was intended as a guide "for the use of those Godly Ladies and Gentlewomen, who are industrious for the improvement of their talent God has given them, in helping their poor sick neighbors" [61].

By the turn of the eighteenth century, bonesetting was commonly performed by laypersons, particularly in England. Sally Mapp, daughter of an English bonesetter whose techniques had been handed down for centuries from one generation to another, drove her carriage from Epsom to London "to take charge of the dislocated limbs of the nobility and gentry" [61].

As the nineteenth century arrived, many medical doctors adopted some of the bonesetters' methods. The luxations and subluxations referred to by Hippocrates, Parè, and other medical practitioners were painful conditions requiring treatment for relief of pain and deformity. However, some medical practitioners felt that slightly misaligned vertebrae could cause organic disease by pinching spinal nerves. In 1842, Dr. J. Evans Riadore, a Fellow of the Royal College of Surgeons, proposed that:

> Every organ and muscle in the body is dependent more or less upon the spinal nerves. . . . When one vertebra forms a slight exception in the regularity of the spinal line, either by height or distance from its fellows, a serious train of nervous symptoms may supervene. [194]

Thus, some physicians were manipulating vertebrae as a treatment for disease more than fifty years before D.D. Palmer "discovered" chiropractic. "Stretch beds" and other mechanotherapy devices were also popular at that time [176].

In 1867, in the *British Medical Journal*, the respected English surgeon Sir James Paget stated that some manipulations performed by bonesetters had value:

> Few of you are likely to practice without having a bone-setter for a rival; and if he can cure a case which you have failed to cure, his fortune may be made and yours marred. . . . Learn, then, to imitate what is good and avoid what is bad in the practice of bone-setters. [61]

In 1871, Wharton Hood, M.D., published *On Bonesetting* and a series of articles on this subject in a British medical journal. "The whole mystery of 'bone-setting,' precisely what it could do and where it was injurious, was laid open to the medical profession in the plainest language," he wrote [61].

Osteopathy's Roots

In 1874, Andrew Taylor Still, the "lightning bonesetter" of Kirksville, Missouri, announced his belief that misaligned joints could interfere with blood supply to cause disease. "The rule of the artery must be absolute," he proposed, "or disease will be the result." Still declared that manipulation of "deranged, displaced bones, nerves, muscles" would remove all obstructions, "thereby setting the machinery of life moving." His autobiography stated:

> I could twist a man one way and cure flux, fever, colds and the diseases of the climate; shake a child and stop scarlet fever, croup, and diphtheria; and cure whooping cough in three days by a wring of the child's neck. [183]

Still also claimed that manipulation could cure 75 percent of appendicitis cases brought to him.

Twenty years previously, at the age of twenty-six, he had assumed the title "Doctor." There is no evidence that he graduated from a medical school. Like most practitioners of his day (physicians as well as bonesetters), he learned from experience, probably from working with his father who was a Methodist minister as well as a physician.

"God is the father of osteopathy," Still wrote in his autobiography, "and I am not ashamed of the child of His mind. . . . He who so forgets God's teachings as to use drugs forfeits the respect of this school and its teachings."

As medical science developed, osteopathy gradually incorporated all of its theories and practices and abandoned Still's dogma [66]. Today, except for additional emphasis on musculoskeletal diagnosis and treatment, the scope of osteopathy is identical to that of medicine. Most osteopaths who use manipulation limit its use to musculoskeletal problems. However, the percentage of practitioners using osteopathic manipulative treatment and the extent of use have both been falling steadily [97]. Some still believe that manipulative treatment encourages the body's natural tendency toward good health, an idea that resembles the thinking of many chiropractors [19].

Palmer's "Big Idea"

Osteopathy's development and the growing popularity of bonesetting created conditions that were ripe for chiropractic's appearance. Chiropractic's founder, D.D. Palmer (1845–1913), emigrated to the United States from Canada at the age of twenty and worked for various periods of time as a schoolmaster, farmer, and grocer. He also became engrossed in medical and psychic practices that were prevalent toward the latter half of the nineteenth century. He dabbled in phrenology and spiritualism and began practicing "magnetic healing" in Burlington, Iowa, in 1886. During the following year, he moved to Davenport, Iowa, rented a suite of rooms, advertised extensively, and developed a thriving practice.

Magnetic healers claimed to transfer healing energy while touching or passing their hands over the patient's body [142:69]. Palmer wrote that his aim was to locate dysfunctional organs and to impart "a life force from his hands, which most patients can feel, into that dominant organ, arousing it to action, thereby assisting it to throw off the unnatural condition" [138]. Ralph Lee Smith, author of *At Your Own Risk*, has described magnetic healing as "a crude form of hypnotism" [173].

In 1895, Palmer announced a "discovery" based on principles nearly identical to those of osteopathy, with which he was familiar. The main difference was that Palmer attributed disease to misaligned vertebrae that pinched spinal nerves, whereas Still held that "disturbed arteries" were responsible. Palmer described chiropractic's seminal event this way in his 1910 textbook, *The Chiropractor's Adjuster:*

> One question was always uppermost in my mind in my search for the cause of disease. I desired to know why one person was ailing and his associate, eating at the same table, working in the same shop, at the same bench, was not. Why? What difference was there in the two persons that caused one to have pneumonia, catarrh, typhoid or rheumatism, while his partner, similarly situated, escaped? Why? This question had worried thousands for centuries and was answered in September, 1895.
>
> Harvey Lillard, a janitor, in the Ryan Block, where I had my office, had been so deaf for 17 years that he could not hear the racket of a wagon on the street or the ticking of a watch. I made inquiry as to the cause of his deafness and was informed that when he was exerting himself in a cramped, stooping position, he felt something give way in his back and immediately became deaf. An examination showed a vertebra racked from its normal position. I reasoned that if that vertebra was replaced, the man's hearing should be restored. With this object in view, a half-hour's talk persuaded Mr. Lillard to allow me to replace it. I racked it into position by using the spinous process as a lever and soon the man could hear as before. There was nothing "accidental" about this, as it was accomplished with an object in view, and the result expected was obtained. There was nothing "crude" about this adjustment; it was specific, so much so that no Chiropractor has equaled it. . . .

Shortly after this relief from deafness, I had a case of heart trouble which was not improving. I examined the spine and found a displaced vertebra pressing against the nerves which innervate the heart. I adjusted the vertebra and gave immediate relief— nothing "accidental" or "crude" about this. Then I began to reason if two diseases, so dissimilar as deafness and heart trouble, came from impingement, a pressure on nerves, were not other disease due to a similar cause? Thus the science (knowledge) and art (adjusting) of Chiropractic were formed at that time. I then began a systematic investigation for the cause of all diseases and have been amply rewarded. [137:18]

It would be interesting to know how Lillard, who was "thoroughly deaf," could carry on a conversation with Palmer. It would also be interesting to know how adjusting a spinal bone could restore hearing when the nerves responsible for hearing are located entirely within the skull. Despite these inconsistencies, and sounding very much like Andrew Taylor Still, D.D. Palmer declared that "95 percent of diseases are caused by displaced vertebrae; the remainder by luxations of other joints." Palmer's new treatment method was named by the Reverend Samuel H. Weed, who suggested the Greek term "Cheir-prakticos," which means "hand practitioner."

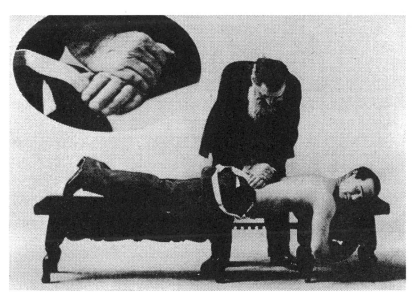

D.D. Palmer delivering a lumbar adjustment.
From B.J. Palmer's *The Science of Chiropractic* (1906).

Early chiropractors maintained that the nervous system described in the anatomy books of their day was a "neurological superstition." According to them, all bodily functions are determined by the flow of "Innate Intelligence" from the brain to the spinal cord and out through the openings between the vertebrae. The "big idea" alleged that removing interference with this flow would enable the body to heal itself.

In 1897, in Davenport, D.D. Palmer opened the Palmer School and Cure, which had a three-week course of study and no entrance requirement other than payment of the tuition. Not long afterward, it was renamed the Palmer Infirmary and Chiropractic Institute. Noting Palmer's activities, the *Journal of Osteopathy* published this observation:

> There is one fake magnetic healer in Iowa who issued a paper devoted to his alleged new system, and who until recently made up his entire publication from the contents of the *Journal of Osteopathy*, changing it only to insert the name of his own practice.

Although Still maintained that disease could be treated by manipulating the joints to remove interference with blood supply, Palmer claimed to be the first to treat the *real* cause of disease by adjusting the vertebrae to remove "nerve interference":

> There is a vast difference between treating effects and adjusting the causes. I was the first to adjust the cause of disease.... The man who had the intellectual capacity to comprehend the displacement of vertebrae; the mental ability to grasp the significance of nerve impingement; the power to conceive and discriminate between normal and abnormal positions; the foresight and wisdom to discern the outcome; the genius of originality to create such a unique science; the judgment needed for the occasion; the brain caliber capable of reasoning on this heretofore perplexing question—the cause of disease; the sense of touch required to discover a racked vertebra and the skill and tact to replace it, was the one destined to discover and develop the science which he named chiropractic. [135]

Both Still and Palmer were wrong in their contentions that slightly misaligned vertebrae would encroach upon blood vessels or nerves in the openings between the vertebrae. In the absence of degenerative changes, there is ample room for spinal nerves and blood vessels. Nevertheless, both osteopathy and chiropractic have not only survived but have prospered. Osteopathy has done so by joining the medical mainstream. Chiropractic, still attached to its cultist roots, has advanced mainly through political maneuvering.

3

From Cult to Profession

Whereas Daniel David Palmer came up with "the big idea" that subluxated vertebrae cause 95 percent of all disease, his son Bartlett Joshua Palmer (1882–1961) was responsible for chiropractic's survival. Ralph Lee Smith, author of *At Your Own Risk*, described "B.J." as a "commercial and public relations genius" [173]. B.J. battled not only to market chiropractic to the public, but also to sell his own version to other chiropractors. He popularized the slogan "Get the Big Idea and All Else Follows" [103]. He declared that the only treatment needed to improve health was a spinal adjustment and that virtually every condition could be treated chiropractically (see box on next page). While the medical profession has made enormous progress by following the rules of science, chiropractic—until recently—has fit the classic definition of a cult ("obsessive devotion to a person, principle, or ideal").

Early Sales Pitches

B.J. Palmer graduated from his father's school in 1902 and became half-owner during the following year. In 1906, he purchased his father's share and published the first of his many similar books, *The Science of Chiropractic: Its Principles and Adjustments*. He also began an aggressive campaign to attract students to the school, which by then was called The Palmer School of Chiropractic. In an essay called "Do You Want a Profession That Has Backbone?" the book stated:

Are you looking for a profession? If so, choose one that is new, up-to-date, is remunerative from the start, practical in every way, progressive, fascinating, will make you prosperous while making others healthy and happy. . . . Several students have borrowed the necessary funds and repaid the debt within a year. One Chiropractor says, "learning Chiropractic is like falling heir to a fortune."

Your Disease

We know where to find the cause of your ailments. There would be perfect action if the human mechanism was in proper position. We make it our special business to adjust any part of the skeletal frame that is displaced and pressing on nerves. Chiropractic corrects the cause of your trouble, then it is only natural, that you should be well. If you have any of the following ailments, stop taking drugs. Come to the Palmer School of Chiropractic Infirmary and have Chiropractic adjust the cause. . . .

Abscesses (any part of the body); Apoplexy; Asthma; Appendicitis; Bright's disease; Brain fever; Bladder troubles; Bronchitis; Cancer (any part of body); Constipation; Cataract; Cholera Morbus; Child Bed Fever; Catarrh; Colic; Consumption (Quick or chronic); Diabetes; Diarrhoea; Dyspepsia; Dysmenorrhea; Dropsy; Dysentery; Deafness; Diphtheria; Emissions; Epilepsy; Eczema; Erysipelas; Female Diseases; Gleet; Fevers (all types); Goitre; Gravel; Gall Stones; Gout; Gastrodynia; Gonorrhea; Hernia (any part of abdomen); Hysteria; Hay Fever; Heart Disease; Heart Burn; Hydrocele; Impotency; Insomnia; Indigestion; Insanity; Jaundice; Kidney Diseases; Liver Diseases; Lost Manhood; LaGrippe; Leucorrhea; Lumbago; Lupus; Mumps; Measles; Malaria Fever; Meningitis; Neuralgia; Nervous Debility; Ovarian Diseases; Pharynigitis [sic]; Palsy; Pleurisy; Paralysis; Pneumonia; Peritonitis; Piles; Quinsy; Rheumatism (any part of body); Rupture; Sarcocele; Sciatica; Spleen; Scrofula; St. Vitus Dance; Spinal Meningitis; Spinal Diseases; Smallpox; Scurvy; Tumors (any part of body); Typhoid; Urinary Diseases; Varicocele; Vertigo; Worms (any kind); Whooping Cough; Womb: (Inflammation of), (Displacement of), (Tumors of), (Polypi of), (Cancer of).

If your disease is not on this list, bear in mind that this chapter is not as large as a medical dictionary.

From B.J. Palmer's *The Science of Chiropractic* (1906), pages 401–404.
Reformatted to fit on one page.

With a small outlay in cash and time you learn one hundred times more of the cause and its adjustment of disease than can be acquired in any medical college in a four-year course, or an osteopathic college in three years. Such being the case does it not look reasonable that it will pay you to investigate? . . . .

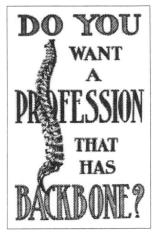

Illustration from B.J. Palmer's 1906 book

The field of common labor is crowded, in Chiropractic there is an increasing demand for those who are qualified. . . .

Chiropractic is American. The cause of disease is comprehensible. Adjustments are readily learned and understood. Every move a chiropractor makes is done with a special aim in view. You are not asked to believe that which is not demonstrated in the clinic. Theory does not enter into its composition, it is based upon deductions from practical, reasonable and actual experience. [136:407]

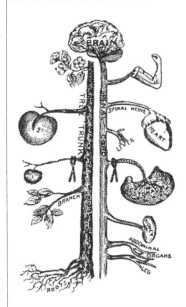

ILLUSTRATION NO. 43.

This illustration represents the trunk, branches and fruit of a tree. The trunk corresponds to the spinal cord, the branches to the nerves, and the fruit to the organs of the human body, as shown in the right half of the cut. Pliers are represented as pinching a limb, also the nerves which control the functions of the stomach, the results are immature worthless fruit, and a diseased stomach.

In the human body, the intervertebral foramina are the pinchers. The vertebrae are wrenched, displaced, occluding the openings thru which the nerves pass. Chiropractors assert that this pressure causes 100 per cent of all diseases. The leaves and fruit are at the twig ends of the limbs. The organs of the body are at the peripheral endings of the spinal nerves. Disturbed functions in any other branch, or spinal nerve, would have shown similar results in other fruit or vital organs.

From B.J. Palmer's *The Science of Chiropractic* (1906)

The book also expressed great hostility toward the medical profession:

> The medical schools arrest progress by binding the people to drug treatments, killing research, forcing idleness upon active brains, branding with iniquity original thinkers who revolt against servile intimidation of the medical code, and refuse to follow their dictates, like sheep, unquestionably. Human health is priceless and far too valuable to jeopardize in the interest of hostile, prejudiced, monopolistic schools. [136:21]

B.J. subsequently commented:

> Our school is on a business, not a professional basis. . . . We manufacture chiropractors. . . . Give me a simple mind that thinks along single tracts, give me 30 days to instruct him, and that individual can go forth on the highways and by ways and get more sick people well than the best, most complete, all around, unlimited medical education of any medical man who ever lived. [133]

Dealing with Competition

During the early 1900s, hundreds of chiropractic schools had sprung up, many of them offering correspondence courses. Competing courses were also offered by practitioners of "spondylotherapy," which was claimed to cure disease by rapidly tapping or percussing the spine. By 1921, the Palmer school had 2,000 students and an annual income of $1 million [80]. Many were veterans of World War I who had been released from the armed forces without an occupation or trade.

In addition to running the school, B.J. conducted a brisk mail-order business, selling chiropractors throughout the nation such items as adjustment tables, miniature spine sections, and portraits of himself [173]. In 1924, with enrollment peaking at 3,000, B.J. introduced the neurocalometer, a heat-detecting device (thermocouple) that, when moved along the spine, was supposed to locate subluxations, even in patients without symptoms. The neurocalometer was presented as infallible for locating "nerve pressure" by measuring differences in temperature between one side of the spine and the other. Palmer maintained that any chiropractor who did not use the neurocalometer was incompetent and could not succeed in practice. He offered his patented instrument for sale for as much as $2,200, but only to graduates of his school.

This blatant commercial pitch caused some of Palmer's closest supporters to desert him and start their own chiropractic colleges.

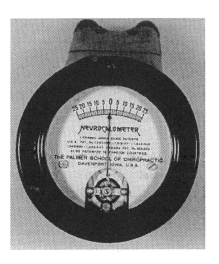

B.J. Palmer claimed that the neurocalometer could locate "subluxations" and "pinched nerves" by comparing the skin temperature over both sides of the spine. The instrument is run along the spine with a probe on each side. A "reading" is considered significant if the needle moves back and forth abruptly over a spinal segment. The original device used a handheld detector connected by a long wire to the meter, which was housed in a solid walnut case. Some chiropractors still use instruments similar to the more "modern" version shown here.

Enrollment at the Palmer School declined. In 1930, Palmer tried again to make the Palmer School of Chiropractic the "only school of chiropractic." He proposed a new theory, that subluxation of the atlas (at the top of the spine) was the primary cause of disease. He informed the profession that chiropractors not schooled in the new adjustive technique required for correction of atlas subluxations were not providing correct treatment. According to Palmer, only chiropractors graduating from the Palmer School, or those who returned to the school for additional training, could successfully treat disease. He called his new technique the "Hole-in-One" ("H.I.O.") treatment. He claimed that correct adjustment of the atlas would cause secondary subluxations in other portions of the spine to "fall into place," correcting the entire spine and removing the cause of 95 percent of all diseases simply by adjusting the spine. This "one-cause, one-cure" concept was the epitome of cultism.

According to Palmer, chiropractors who had been taught that misalignment of certain vertebrae caused certain diseases would be "out of date" unless they took additional training in the H.I.O. technique at his school, where students were not permitted to adjust below the atlas. The H.I.O. theory was so contrary to Palmer's previous teachings that most chiropractors found it even less acceptable than his neurocalometer promotion. Nevertheless, the Palmer School continued to teach H.I.O. technique until 1949, when B.J. reinstated full-spine techniques and extended the course of instruction to four years [191]. Even today, some chiropractors are dedicated to Palmer's upper cervical technique. Many of these belong to the International Upper Cervical Chiropractic Association [188].

Palmer instilled in his students the faith and enthusiasm necessary to sell a controversial service or product. Students have to work like machinery, he said in 1920 [60:89] and again in 1950 [80], "a course of salesmanship goes along with their training."

Widespread Diversity

Whereas the Palmer School advocated the "Hole-in-One" adjustment at the top of the spine, the Logan Basic College of Chiropractic, founded in 1935, taught that sacral misalignment at the *bottom* of the spine was responsible for all the problems above that level. Sacro-occipital technique, developed in 1925, involved manipulation of both ends of the spine.

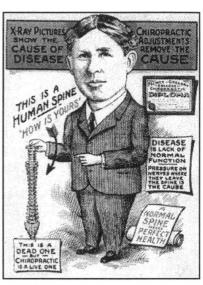

This chiropractor's immodest business card from the 1920s also promised "no drugs, no knife."

Many chiropractic methods evolved from Palmer's theory of vertebral misalignment. One of the most popular was the Parker system in which a full-spine x-ray was used to measure millimeters of vertebral displacement up and down the spine to determine the number of spinal adjustments needed [140].

In the meric system, certain vertebrae corresponded to certain organs. To effect a cure, it was only necessary to adjust a vertebra corresponding to a diseased organ. If a person had kidney trouble, for example, the chiropractor would adjust the 10th or the 11th thoracic vertebra, which was designated as "the kidney place."

A 1947 chiropractic textbook published by the National College of Chiropractic, a mixer college that moved from Davenport to Chicago in 1908, offered these "clinical facts":

> In nearly all affections involving the structures of the head and face, such as the ear, eye, nose, and throat, subluxations exist, and that, moreover, adjustment of subluxated vertebrae is followed by a cure or improvement of such disease. . . . The tenth dorsal vertebra is found subluxated in all cases of kidney diseases. . . . The second lumbar vertebra is virtually always found subluxated in constipation.

. . . A subluxation in the fifth and sixth cervical segments . . . markedly alters the normal conditions of the tonsils, and they then become a favorable medium for the entrance of this specific infection [rheumatic infection]. This same principle applies to all infectious and contagious diseases. [93]

Spinal adjustments were also touted as a preventive measure. The National College of Chiropractic, for example, taught:

When a subluxation is produced in the lower dorsal or upper lumbar region of the vertebral column, no untoward effects may follow at once. But years later, perhaps, the individual develops typhoid fever. [93]

Opposition to Immunization

B.J. Palmer called vaccination a form of "poisoning" [136:17]. Persistent devotion to his dogma was exemplified in the 1950s when the National Chiropractic Association campaigned against polio vaccination during an epidemic and recommended chiropractic adjustments for preventing and treating the disease. An article in the association's March 1959 journal offered this advice:

The test tube fight against polio has failed. . . . The death rate has increased among the children who have been vaccinated. . . . There is no vaccine against fatigue or a traumatic lesion in the anterior cord or motor cells. . . . In the mild, and especially in the more acute chiropractic is supreme. Adjustments of the entire spine will break up the cord congestion, if given within the three days of grace given by Nature. Chiropractic aids nature . . . . The fatigue lesion of acute polio can be caused by other factors, such as whooping cough and smallpox vaccines. The latter can cause vaccinosyphilis in the pure blood of children. Acute polio will take place with paralysis on the same side the vaccination is given; that is, in cases of vaccino-poliomyelitis. [63]

Responding to various attacks on the polio vaccine, the U.S. Surgeon General defended its use and effectiveness:

During the three and one-half years [the Salk vaccine] has been in use, the effectiveness rate of 60 to 90 percent has been consistently maintained. Nor is there any evidence that properly vaccinated persons are losing their immunity and becoming more susceptible to polio. [32]

Although most chiropractors today do not openly campaign against vaccination, and a few even support it, chiropractic theory still fosters opposition to any form of artificial immunization [43,131]. The World Chiropractic Alliance, a small group of straight chiropractors, actively opposes immunization [37], while the American Chiropractic Association, recognizing that vaccination has been shown to be a cost-effective and clinically effective procedure for certain viral and microbial diseases, does not support compulsory vaccination. Its current policy is to support "each individual's right to freedom of choice in his/her own health care based on an informed awareness of the benefits and possible adverse effects of vaccination" [1].

• **Medicine** - No scientific basis - a dangerous guardian of the public health.

• **Chiropractic** - The answer to the cause of disease and natural immunity.

• **Vaccinations** - More harm than good.

• **Mandatory Vaccination** - Totally unconstitutional.

Message in an anti-immunization booklet from the 1970s [177].

A former president of the International Chiropractic Association said in 1993: "I am a firm opponent of artificial immunization and the antiquated germ theory on which it is based" [16].

In a 1997 issue of *Today's Chiropractic*, a chiropractic author advises that "When chiropractors embrace vaccination, they are turning their backs on their philosophy, on their purpose, on their reason for being" [113].

Straights vs. Mixers

D.D. Palmer's theory that vertebral misalignment causes 95 percent of all diseases and that spinal adjustment is the only treatment needed to cure or prevent disease did not allow for the use of other treatment methods. It was inevitable, however, that some chiropractors would want to include heat, cold, colonic irrigation, and other measures that Palmer considered unnecessary and outside the scope of chiropractic.

In 1905, the Minnesota American Chiropractic Association was formed to support and promote the use of additional treatment methods. This was the beginning of the "war" between "mixer" chiropractors, who wanted to include other treatment methods, and "straight" chiropractors, who believed that only spinal adjustments were needed to cure disease. D.D. Palmer said of the Minnesota group:

They have mixed what little they know of this science [chiropractic] with medicinal and mechanical remedies, until today, there is but little, if any, resemblance between what is called chiropractic in Minnesota and that which is taught at the Palmer School. [103]

In 1906, B.J. Palmer formed the Universal Chiropractic Association to combat the mixer policies of the Minnesota group, to seek licensure of chiropractors, and to provide legal defense for chiropractors who practiced "straight chiropractic."

The theory of vertebral misalignment as a cause of disease proved to be appealing to laypersons. Public pressure to license chiropractors increased. The first laws to legalize chiropractic were passed in Kansas in 1913 and in North Dakota in 1915.

Subluxation theories even attracted the attention and support of a few medical practitioners. One was a Harvard Medical School graduate named Alfred Walton, M.D. In 1915, Walton published a brochure called "Chiropractic" in order to "awaken an interest in the new Science of Chiropractic." He stated:

> The condition of the spine is the keynote of the entire situation; if a careful digital and visual examination of the spine is made, it will reveal all the patient complains of, which results in a great saving of time, as an examination of the spine reveals the actual cause of 95% of all diseases, therefore, why should it be necessary to concern oneself with a minute study of effects? What is to be gained?
>
> If the cause of a serious interference with the function of the kidneys be due to a lower thoracic vertebra being out of alignment, from the standpoint of the clinician, does it make any material difference whether the pathological changes are of chronic interstitial nephritis, or whether it be chronic parenchymatous nephritis? Adjustments require but a fraction of the time we now spend in investigating symptoms. [194]

In 1926, B.J. Palmer founded the Chiropractic Health Bureau, a straight chiropractic organization, which became the International Chiropractic Association (ICA) in 1941. In 1928, the National Chiropractic Association (NCA) was formed to support the mixer policies of chiropractors who had split off from Palmer's straight chiropractic.

The appearance of the NCA intensified the war between straight chiropractors who were faithful to the Palmer School and the mixer chiropractors who wanted to include other therapies. In 1958, B.J. Palmer, supporting straight chiropractic and denouncing mixed chiropractic, said of the National Chiropractic Association:

The NCA is fully cognizant of what they do. They know they are destroying everything Chiropractic except its name. . . . The ICA, by contrast, is an organization composed of Chiropractors, whose programs, speakers, legislative and legal intentions are to preserve, protect, defend and make possible everything pro-chiropractic and nothing pro-medical. [133]

Claude O. Watkins, D.C., a 1925 Palmer graduate who crusaded for educational reform and served as NCA board chairman during the early 1940s, commented on chiropractic factionalism in a remarkably candid report he issued in 1944:

Dr. D.D. Palmer discovered the subluxation of the vertebra and evolved the theory of nerve interference. He tested this knowledge and from it grew the science of chiropractic. First, new types of manipulative methods were added. Then other physical methods of treatment were developed until today modern chiropractic embraces many methods and theories as do all other branches of science. In the early history of chiropractic the leaders developed what they called a philosophy of chiropractic but which served more as a doctrine. This "doctrine" was supposed to be invulnerable and to be subscribed to much as one subscribes to a religious faith. These early leaders, apparently for purposes of self-aggrandizement, insisted that their methods were the alpha and omega of chiropractic. . . . Indeed, due to the lack of scientific organization to synthesize manipulative methods several systems and cults have developed, each specializing in its particular system. [192]

By 1950, forty-four states had passed chiropractic licensing laws. To comply with these laws, the Palmer School lengthened its course of instruction from eighteen months to four years. With an increase in school time, there was a greater emphasis on salesmanship. "We teach them the idea and then show them how to sell it," B.J. Palmer explained. His motto "Early to bed, early to rise, work like hell, and advertise" was painted on the wall of the Palmer School [12]. Still promoting the Hole-in-One theory in 1959, B.J. Palmer advised the chiropractic profession:

The primary, causative vertebral subluxation can be only where there are no intervertebral osseous locks, viz., between occiput, atlas, and axis, except for the odontoid which prevents one direction only. The only place a causative vertebral subluxation can be adjusted is in that area. [135]

In 1963, the NCA became the American Chiropractic Association (ACA). Today, both the ACA and the ICA promote use of the spinal adjustment for "restoring and maintaining health." And, as was the case in 1905, the ACA supports use of a greater variety of treatment methods while the ICA remains faithful to Palmer's version of straight chiropractic. Both groups embrace a broad scope of practice, offering a limited treatment method based on adjustment of vertebral subluxations.

Some chiropractic colleges still teach straight chiropractic, and licensing laws vary from state to state. Despite inconsistencies in what chiropractors do, the chiropractic profession has managed to grow and to gain professional status. Today, with more chiropractors practicing mixed chiropractic than straight chiropractic, the membership of the ACA greatly outnumbers that of the ICA.

Increased Insurance Coverage

In 1968, the Department of Health, Education, and Welfare recommended against chiropractic inclusion in the Medicare program. In a report to Congress, it concluded that "the chiropractor's approach to health and disease is radically different from that of osteopathy and medicine" and that chiropractic's educational system was inadequate [42]. (See Chapter 5.)

Nevertheless, in 1972, Congress responded to a flood of letters and telegrams by adding chiropractic coverage for manual adjustment of the spine to correct "subluxations demonstrated by x-ray to exist" [175]. Other federal programs offering chiropractic coverage use a similar limitation. In January 2000, x-ray examination of chiropractic Medicare patients will no longer be mandatory, but the definition of chiropractic will not change.

Because insurance companies generally balked at the idea of covering chiropractic services, chiropractors have also lobbied aggressively to force them to do so. Today, forty-six states have "insurance equality" laws and virtually all major health insurance carriers cover chiropractic care for musculoskeletal problems. In all fifty states, the District of Columbia, the Virgin Islands, and Puerto Rico, chiropractic services are authorized by the State Worker's Compensation programs.

Academic Recognition

In 1974, the Council on Chiropractic Education (CCE), established by the National Chiropractic Association in 1947, gained recognition by the U.S. Office of Education, making it possible to encourage upgrading of chiropractic colleges. Today, all sixteen chiropractic colleges are accredited by the CCE. Graduation from a CCE-accredited school is required for licensure of chiropractors in most states. But such accreditation has not curbed teaching of D.D. Palmer's subluxation theory and has not eliminated the nonsense often associated with some forms of chiropractic treatment.

Less Medical Opposition

In the 1960s, the American Medical Association formed a Committee on Quackery whose primary mission was to contain and then eliminate chiropractic as a recognized healthcare service. In November 1966, the AMA House of Delegates adopted a resolution stating (in part):

> Chiropractic is an unscientific cult whose practitioners lack the necessary training and background to diagnose and treat human disease. Chiropractic constitutes a hazard to rational health care in the United States because of the substandard and unscientific education of its practitioners and their rigid adherence to an irrational, unscientific approach to disease causation. . . .
> Patients should entrust their health care only to those who have a broad scientific knowledge of diseases and ailments of all kinds, and who are capable of diagnosing and treating them with all the resources of modern medicine. The delay of proper medical care caused by chiropractors and their opposition to the many scientific advances in modern medicine, such as lifesaving vaccines, often ends with tragic results.

In 1976, various chiropractors began a series of lawsuits charging that the AMA and others had conspired to destroy chiropractic and to illegally deprive chiropractors of access to laboratory, x-ray, and hospital facilities. Most of the defendant groups agreed in out-of-court settlements that their physician members were free to decide for themselves how to deal with chiropractors. In 1980, the AMA revised its principles of medical ethics along the same lines and did not include the "cult" label in the revision. Nevertheless, in 1987, a federal court judge ruled that the AMA had engaged in an illegal boycott.

Many chiropractors represent the ruling as an endorsement of chiropractic, but it was not. The judge concluded that the AMA had good reason to criticize chiropractors but should not have attempted to contain and eliminate an entire licensed profession without first demonstrating that a less restrictive campaign could not protect the public. She stated:

All of the parties to the case, including the plaintiffs and the AMA, agreed that chiropractic treatment of diseases such as diabetes, high blood pressure, cancer, heart disease and infectious disease is not proper, and that the historic theory of chiropractic that there is a single cause and cure of disease was wrong. . . . There was evidence that the chiropractic theory of subluxations was unscientific, and evidence that some chiropractors engaged in unscientific practices. [65]

Although the antitrust ruling does not bar the AMA or anyone else from legitimately criticizing chiropractic, professional organizations have been very reluctant to do so.

Partial Scientific Support

Despite failing to prove or discard the vertebral subluxation theory, the chiropractic profession has gained status because spinal manipulation can be useful for treating mechanical-type back and neck pain. During the 1990s, reports by RAND [49,165] and the Agency for Health Care Policy and Research [27] endorsed limited use of spinal manipulation (not chiropractic), thereby boosting the image of chiropractors (who do most of the manipulating). But many chiropractors have misrepresented these reports as a general endorsement of chiropractic treatment [26,162,187].

Practice Guidelines

In 1992, showing signs of professional maturity, a consensus conference commissioned by the Congress of Chiropractic State Associations attempted to establish quality assurance guidelines for chiropractic practice [71]. The resultant document, called the Mercy Guidelines, did not adequately condemn questionable chiropractic diagnostic and treatment methods (such as moire topography and instrument adjusting), and it did little to change the theory and practice of chiropractic. Many chiropractors rejected the Mercy Guidelines, since most chiropractors felt that any restrictions placed on the practice of chiropractic were unacceptable. In fact, a panel representing straight chiropractors produced guidelines for subluxation-based chiropractors [146]. Thus, while educational requirements in chiropractic colleges have been raised, and spinal manipulation is gaining recognition as a treatment for some types of back pain, the chiropractic profession continues to be guided by the subluxation theory.

Serious Problems Remain

With increasing acceptance of the use of spinal manipulation for treating mechanical-type back and neck pain, greater attention will be focused on the work of chiropractors, most of whom use manipulation to "restore and maintain health" as well as to relieve back and neck pain.

In October 1998, the *New England Journal of Medicine* published the results of two well-designed studies that tested long-held chiropractic beliefs. One found that adding chiropractic manipulation to standard medical care provided no benefit to children with mild or moderate asthma [15]. The other compared the use of physical therapy, chiropractic manipulation, and instruction with an educational booklet for treating low-back pain without sciatica. This study found that physical therapy and chiropractic manipulation had similar effects and costs and that patients receiving these treatments had only marginally better outcomes than those receiving the minimal intervention of an educational booklet [35].

An editorial in the same issue of the journal stated that "for some musculoskeletal conditions, chiropractic care does provide some benefit to patients." However, the author concluded that there is little evidence to support spinal manipulation for nonmusculoskeletal conditions and that it is inappropriate to consider chiropractic as a broad-based alternative to traditional medical care [163].

A month later, the *Journal of the American Medical Association* attacked another widely held chiropractic belief. It published a study whose authors concluded that neck manipulation "does not seem to have a positive effect on episodic tension-type headache" [30].

As chiropractic gains status as a profession, it will be held more accountable for what its practitioners say and do. Although the chiropractic profession has come a long way in shedding its image as a cult, it has not yet renounced or abandoned the cultist tenets upon which it is based. Many chiropractors still cling tightly to Palmer dogma, and many more promote spinal adjustments for "restoring and maintaining health." The remaining chapters of this book provide the information needed to make informed decisions about chiropractic care.

4

The "Subluxation" Issue

To understand chiropractic, it is vital to understand what "subluxation" means. This is not simple to pin down. Medical doctors and chiropractors define the term differently. The medical meaning is incomplete or partial dislocation—a condition, visible on x-ray films, in which the bony surfaces of a joint no longer face each other exactly but remain partially aligned. Chiropractors define subluxations in many ways and cannot agree among themselves about what they are, how they should be diagnosed, how they should be treated, or even what they should be called. Nearly three hundred alternative names have been proposed [152].

Craig Nelson, D.C., an associate professor at Northwestern College of Chiropractic, has aptly summarized the chiropractic spectrum of beliefs:

> The concept of the subluxation is simultaneously chiropractic's central defining clinical principle and the source of contentious debate and disagreement within the profession. As chiropractic has evolved . . . one faction of the profession has distanced itself from the original subluxation theory as formulated by D.D. Palmer. . . . In the main, this faction . . . has concluded that subluxations as Palmer imagined them simply do not exist.
>
> At the same time, a large faction of believers (both individuals and institutions) within the profession still cling to undiluted Palmerism; those who characterize themselves and their beliefs as subluxation-based. While some of Palmer's explanations regarding mechanisms may have been modified to accommodate a more sophisticated understanding of physiology and pathology, this

31

faction of the profession remains steadfast in its belief that spinal subluxations represent a critical factor (*the* critical factor?) in human health and disease.

There is also a middle ground. While some institutions no longer make direct appeals to subluxation and eschew the use of the term itself, many of the policies and principles they advocate are predicated and inspired by subluxation theory. For example, the admonition to the public, made almost universally by the profession, that they should have a chiropractor evaluate their spinal health even when they are [symptom-free] relies solely on subluxation theory for its validity. The way students are taught in all chiropractic colleges to locate, evaluate, and adjust specific vertebral segments is an expression of subluxation doctrine. And the belief, widely if not universally held, that spinal dysfunction can have effects beyond simply producing back pain owes itself to subluxation theory. [130]

Before elaborating on what chiropractors think and do about subluxations, let's discuss some pertinent facts about the body.

Spinal Function

The spine (backbone) is composed of twenty-six vertebrae that have 103 joints connecting the vertebrae to each other and to the ribs, the skull, and the pelvis. Twenty-three disks serve as cushions between the vertebra. Twenty-six pairs of spinal nerves exit between the vertebrae, and five pairs exit through sacral openings. The bony arches of the vertebrae encircle and protect the spinal cord and nerves.

D.D. Palmer originally announced that spinal misalignments ("subluxations") cause the nearby nerves to develop abnormal "tone" (tension) that causes the body to become ill. A few years later, he declared that health depends on a steady flow of "Innate Intelligence" or "nerve energy" throughout the nervous system and that even slight misalignments can hinder this flow. B.J. Palmer subsequently proclaimed that spinal misalignments pinch nerves as they exit the spine between the vertebrae. Both taught that the nervous system is the master controller of the body and that spinal "adjustments" can correct nearly all types of health problems.

These ideas do not correspond to scientific knowledge of anatomy, physiology, or pathology. The nervous system is not the "master" of all bodily functions. Hormones, enzymes, other circulating chemicals, immune reactions, and countless autonomous reactions inside the body's cells play important roles in health and in defense against disease. Moreover, it has never been demonstrated that spinal misalignments cause disease elsewhere in the body, that chiropractic "adjustments" can realign the spine, or that "pinched nerves" have any effect on general health. Nor has anyone demonstrated that nerves are prone to pinching as they exit between the vertebrae. In fact, as illustrated by the figure below, there is ample room at the point of exit.

The brain, spinal cord, and spinal nerves are not in direct contact with the vertebrae but are surrounded by protective membranes. The nerves exit through bony channels that are padded with blood vessels and fatty tissue. Twenty-five years ago, Edmund S. Crelin, Ph.D., a prominent anatomist at Yale University, demonstrated with cadavers that twisting the spine does not cause impingement unless the force applied is so great that it would disable or kill a living person [51]. (See Appendix B.)

Even if minor pinching could occur, its effect would be insignificant. Neurophysiologic research has demonstrated that a nerve impulse travels more slowly in an area of partial compression but resumes normal flow beyond the affected area. In other words, partial blockage has no significant effect on function. Complete blockage of sensory impulses intended for the

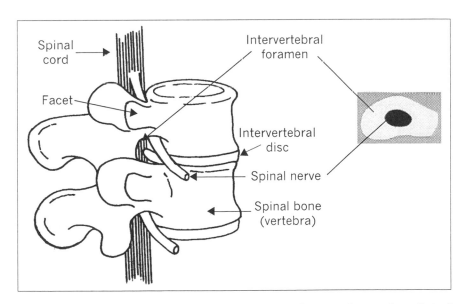

Spinal cord

Facet

Intervertebral foramen

Intervertebral disc

Spinal nerve

Spinal bone (vertebra)

Normally there is ample room for spinal nerves to pass between the vertebrae. Spinal nerves are rarely pinched or irritated unless there is a protruding disc, bony spur, other degenerative condition, or tumor that causes encroachment. The right-hand drawing compares the diameter of a nerve and the opening (foramen) through which it passes.

brain would cause loss of feeling in the affected body part. Skin changes such as dryness would also occur. Complete blockage of nerve impulses to a muscle would result in paralysis. The specific changes would be predictable based on scientific knowledge of neuroanatomy. For example, if the spinal cord were severed below the fourth cervical vertebra, the spinal nerves would be shut off. Paralysis and loss of sensation would occur in musculoskeletal structures from the neck down, but the body's organs would continue to function. Since spinal nerves supply the sphincter muscles of the bladder and the anus, bladder and bowel control would be lost.

Partial displacement of a spinal bone occurs in a *spondylolisthesis*, a condition that is usually congenital, usually causes no symptoms, and is not correctable by any form of chiropractic treatment. Because the ligaments connecting the spinal bones are quite strong, vertebral dislocations rarely occur after birth and are unlikely without severe injury that would require surgical treatment, not manipulation. Herniated disks, arthritic joint changes, tumors, bony overgrowths, and other degenerative changes of the spine can interfere with nerve function. However, these problems do not cause disease in remote organs and are not correctable by spinal manipulation. When more significant compression occurs, the most common effects are pain, numbness, feelings of pins and needles, decreased reflexes, and/or weakness or paralysis of the muscles served by the affected nerves. Most conditions in which nerves are actually compressed are not appropriate for treatment with manipulation.

Even if the nervous system were the dominant factor in determining health, chiropractors would have access to only part of it. The brain itself and the twelve pairs of cranial nerves (including those related to sight, hearing, breathing, heart function, and digestion) exit through the base of the skull and are not accessible to manipulation. The nerves exiting from the sacrum are also inaccessible to manipulation. Appendix A includes a more detailed analysis issued in 1963 by the College of Physicians and Surgeons of the Province of Quebec.

"Modern" Concepts

Many chiropractors still describe subluxations as "bones out of place" and/or "pinched nerves," but the majority speak about "fixations" or other alterations in joint mobility. In 1972, after Congress amended Medicare to cover "manual manipulation of the spine to correct a subluxation (demonstrated by x-ray to exist)" chiropractic leaders met in Houston to

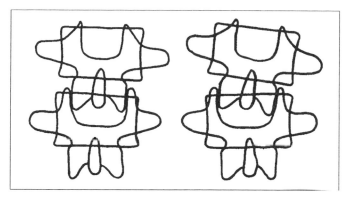

These schematic drawings illustrate the Houston conferees' conception of normally positioned vertebrae (on the left) and a "lateral flexion malposition subluxation characterized by lateral wedging of the disc interspace produced by approximation of the vertebral bodies on the side toward which the vertebra is flexed." Such "misalignments" are not significant unless accompanied by pain and restricted movement.

develop a professionwide definition that would enable chiropractors to get paid. After meeting for two days, the conferees defined "subluxation" as "the alteration of the normal dynamics, anatomical, or physiological relationships of contiguous articular structures" [159]. Their classification system, published as an eight-page insert in the January 1975 *ACA Journal of Chiropractic*, described the supposed x-ray appearance of eighteen types of "subluxations," including "flexion malposition," "extension malposition," "lateral flexion malposition," "rotational malposition," "hypomobility" (also called "fixation subluxation"), "hypermobility," "aberrant motion," "altered interosseous spacing," "foraminal occlusion," scoliosis, and several conditions in which "gross displacements" are evident. Some of these terms are fancy names for the minor degenerative changes that occur as people age; they often have nothing to do with a patient's symptoms and are not changed by chiropractic treatment. Some, as acknowledged in the report itself, are actually not visible on x-ray films. "Altered interosseous spacing," which is very common, is usually the result of disk degeneration, which is not a problem unless the disk herniates. Overall, the classification system enables chiropractors to label common misalignments as "subluxations" responsible for whatever symptoms their patients have.

Entire books have been written about subluxations, and two chiropractic journals are dedicated to subluxation-based research. In *The Neurodynamics of the Vertebral Subluxation* (1977), A.E. Homewood, B.T.A., LL.B., D.P.T., D.C., N.D., F.I.C.C., a former president of two chiropractic colleges, echoed previous teachings that the cause of all disease is "irritation of a mechanical, chemical, or mental nature, alone or in any percentage of combination . . . sufficient to overcome the normal resistance of the body." Citing D.D. Palmer's idea that "auto-suggestion" can cause subluxations, he devoted an entire chapter to discussing how mental stress (psychic irritation) can produce subluxations and vice-versa [79].

Robert A. Leach, D.C., author of *The Chiropractic Theories: A Synopsis of Scientific Research* (1986), states that "many subluxations are 'fixations' in which the vertebrae are locked within their normal range of motion" and that these "can give rise to abnormal somatoautonomic as well as somatosomatic reflexes, by bombarding dorsal horn cells with afferent impulses." He also suggests:

> Abnormal reflexes can set in motion a wide variety of abnormal pathological and functional processes including such conditions as asthma, bronchitis, acute pulmonary atelectasis, muscular atrophy and degeneration, gastrointestinal complaints, coronary artery disease, and pain actually referred to any portion of the body. It is suggested that further clinical research is warranted and that the [somatoautonomic reflex] hypothesis may be the most logical justification for the use of chiropractic adjustment for conditions other than pain syndromes. [115]

The American Chiropractic Association states:

> The most characteristic aspect of chiropractic practice is the correction (reduction) of a subluxated vertebral or pelvic segment(s) by means of making a specific, predetermined adjustment. The purpose of this correction and its determination is to normalize the relationships of segments within their articular surfaces and relieve any attendant neurological, muscular, and vascular disturbances. [9]

In 1996, in an attempt to "unify" chiropractic terminology, the Association of Chiropractic Colleges adopted the following definition:

> A subluxation is a complex of functional and/or structural and/or pathological articular changes that compromise neural integrity and may influence organ system function and general health. A subluxation is evaluated, diagnosed and managed through the use of chiropractic procedures based on the best available rational and empirical evidence.

Referring to this paragraph, a 1997 pamphlet from the Foundation for Chiropractic Education and Research (FCER) explains:

What the above means is that a subluxation is a joint problem (whether a problem with the way the joint is functioning, a physical problem with the joint, or a combination of any of these) that affects the function of nerves and can therefore affect the body's organs and general health.

Chiropractors believe that if joints function properly nerves will function properly and the body will be able to keep itself healthy. [156]

The above definitions, though meaningless, assume that chiropractic subluxations exist and are a common cause of ill health. Some literature written for chiropractors uses such complicated jargon to describe the workings of the nervous system that no one, including chiropractors, can understand it. Some "straight" chiropractors (sometimes referred to as "super-straights") believe that medical diagnosis is unimportant and that their only function should be to "remove subluxations and get the body well." The simple truth, however, is that the vast majority of spinal problems do not affect the body's organs or general health.

FCER has also published a 36-page booklet called "The Role of Subluxations in Chiropractic" [155]. Its notable passages include:

Greater than one hundred terms have been proposed to replace the chiropractic subluxation. Changing the name when referring to the manipulable subluxation—whether to manipulable lesion, neurobiomechanical lesion or orthospondylodysarthric lesion is no more helpful than calling it a spinal "boo boo," an adjustment-seeking lesion, or saying that bad things happen to the spine.— Meridel I. Gatterman, D.C., M.Ed., Dean of Clinical and Chiropractic Science, Western States Chiropractic College.

Subluxation goes beyond metaphor; it is at the heart of chiropractic. This being the case, we must follow where our studies take us, never fearing to modify our core beliefs even when it affects market share or reflects poorly upon our science. . . . Science is mutable; it changes with new data. So, too, does the chiropractic profession. Efforts to better define and understand the subluxation can only help but take us into a brighter future—Dana J. Lawrence, D.C., F.I.C.C., National College of Chiropractic.

Considerable evidence exists to support our conceptual model of subluxation and the philosophical paradigm within which we view that model as reasonable, scientifically valid and clinically profound—Gerald W. Clum, D.C., President, Life Chiropractic College West.

OCTOBER IS SPINAL HEALTH MONTH
PROCLAMATION

Whereas doctors of chiropractic throughout the United States are active during October in a special community health program to improve the spinal health of our citizens; and

Whereas spinal integrity makes it possible for all the organs in the body to function most efficiently; and

Whereas spinal health is essential to proper growth and development; and

Whereas millions of citizens are suffering from numerous illnesses and are unaware that these conditions may be related directly to spinal defects; and

Whereas periodic chiropractic examinations can reveal spinal defects or distortions; and

Whereas increased awareness of the need for spinal health through chiropractic care can correct many illnesses which occur in other parts of the body; and

Whereas poor spinal health costs our nation time, money and manpower; and

Whereas conversely, spinal health assures our nation a more efficient and productive citizenry; and

Whereas the attention of every individual must be brought to the benefits of spinal health and the need for periodic chiropractic examinations; and

Whereas the science of chiropractic and the doctors who practice it have contributed greatly to better health of our citizenry by providing this specialized health care; now

THERFORE, be it resolved that the (city of) (state of) officially joins with the (state) Chiropractic Association in proclaiming the month of October as Spinal Health Month, and urges that this period be dedicated to informing-the citizens of the great (city) (state) of the health benefits of spinal integrity. The (city of) (state of) further commends the doctors of chiropractic and the colleges of chiropractic for their efforts in the public's behalf, and specifically the doctors of chiropractic of this (city) (state) for the community service programs.

Signed _____

Date _____

In 1993, the *ACA Journal of Chiropractic* suggested distributing this model proclamation to governors, mayors, congressional representatives and "all elected or public health officials in your area" [8].

The Vertebral Subluxation Complex (VSC) embraces the holistic nature of the human body, including health, well-being, and the doctor/patient relationship as well as the changes in nerve, muscle, connective, and vascular tissues which are understood to accompany the kinesiologic aberrations of spinal articulations — Anthony L. Rosner, Ph.D., FCER Director of Research.

In 1980, a chiropractic educator asked one thousand chiropractors on the American Chiropractic Association's mailing list whether they agreed with various statements related to Palmerian beliefs. Of 268 respondents, only 4 percent replied that "the chiropractic subluxation is the cause of all disease," but 70 percent said that "the chiropractic subluxation may be related to the cause of most disease." Only 14 percent checked "I do not believe that the chiropractic subluxation is a significant cause of disease." When asked to indicate "the degree of importance you believe subluxation plays," 94 percent checked "50%" or higher for musculoskeletal problems, and 78 percent checked "50%" or more for visceral disease problems [148]. Had members of the International Chiropractors Association or other "straight" chiropractic groups been asked the same questions, their responses would have shown greater degrees of belief in subluxation theory. If such a survey were repeated today, I believe that the subluxation-belief percentages would be smaller but still substantial.

Fitting the Practice to the "Definition"

Since subluxations are "defined" so vaguely, chiropractic is also vaguely defined. One chiropractic college, for example, describes chiropractic's purpose as "the care and treatment of humans without the use of prescription drugs or operative surgery and with special emphasis upon the promotion of neurobiomechanical harmony" [203].

Chiropractic licensing laws reflect the definitional hodgepodge. In 1996, only ten contained the word "subluxation," but twenty (including three with a subluxation phrase) mentioned removing interference to the flow of nerve energy. A few laws stated that chiropractic practice included correcting malposition or misalignment of the vertebrae, and some mentioned adjustment or manipulation of the spine to restore or maintain health. Rhode Island permitted chiropractors to use spinal adjustment, corrective orthopedics and dietetics "for the elimination of the cause of disease." Five states authorized chiropractors to do what is taught in chiropractic schools, and several enabled them to use "chiropractic methods" so long as they did not use prescription drugs or surgery [28]. Most of the laws are so vague that they enable chiropractors to apply the term "subluxation" to any condition—real or imagined—that they would like to treat.

In 1986, the U.S. Department of Health and Human Services' Office of the Inspector General reported on telephone discussions with 145 of 200 chiropractors randomly selected from lists provided from insurance carriers. The report stated that chiropractic manipulation had been the ninth most frequently billed procedure under Medicare Part B during 1983. Referring to the classification system developed at the 1972 Houston consensus conference, the report concluded:

> The Medicare Carriers Manual . . . presents a system for classifying subluxations . . . and a system for relating various symptoms to a particular area of the spine. The manual also lists examples of conditions for which manual manipulation of the spine is not an appropriate treatment. Some critics have suggested that this system has provided a blueprint for chiropractors to work backward to identify the appropriate location of a subluxation for billing purposes, as opposed to treating and billing for a subluxation which has been identified on an x-ray. [126]

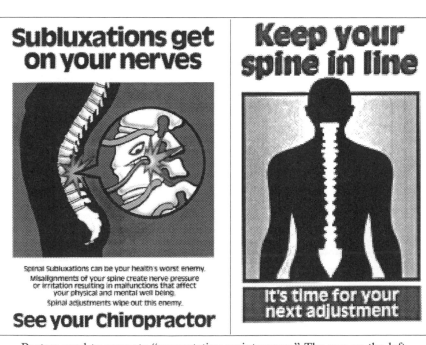

Posters used to promote "preventative maintenance." The one on the left made its debut in 1984. Both are still marketed and used today.

CHART OF EFFECTS OF SPINAL MISALIGNMENTS

"The nervous system controls and coordinates all organs and structures of the human body." (*Gray's Anatomy*, 29th Ed., page 4.) Misalignments of spinal vertebrae and discs may cause irritation to the nervous system and affect the structures, organs, and functions which may result in the conditions shown below.

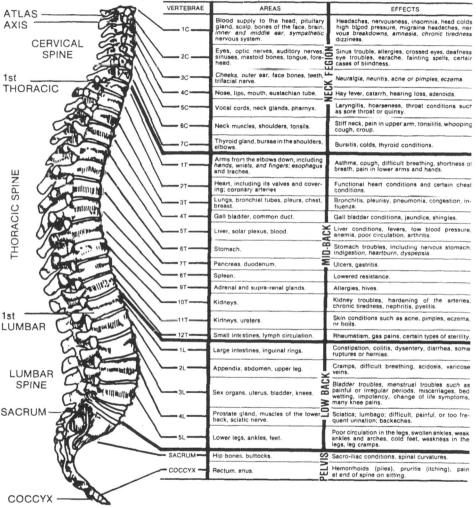

VERTEBRAE	AREAS	EFFECTS
1C	Blood supply to the head, pituitary gland, scalp, bones of the face, brain, inner and middle ear, sympathetic nervous system.	Headaches, nervousness, insomnia, head colds, high blood pressure, migraine headaches, nervous breakdowns, amnesia, chronic tiredness, dizziness.
2C	Eyes, optic nerves, auditory nerves, sinuses, mastoid bones, tongue, forehead.	Sinus trouble, allergies, crossed eyes, deafness, eye troubles, earache, fainting spells, certain cases of blindness.
3C	Cheeks, outer ear, face bones, teeth, trifacial nerve.	Neuralgia, neuritis, acne or pimples, eczema.
4C	Nose, lips, mouth, eustachian tube.	Hay fever, catarrh, hearing loss, adenoids.
5C	Vocal cords, neck glands, pharynx.	Laryngitis, hoarseness, throat conditions such as sore throat or quinsy.
6C	Neck muscles, shoulders, tonsils.	Stiff neck, pain in upper arm, tonsilitis, whooping cough, croup.
7C	Thyroid gland, bursae in the shoulders, elbows.	Bursitis, colds, thyroid conditions.
1T	Arms from the elbows down, including hands, wrists, and fingers; esophagus and trachea.	Asthma, cough, difficult breathing, shortness of breath, pain in lower arms and hands.
2T	Heart, including its valves and covering; coronary arteries.	Functional heart conditions and certain chest conditions.
3T	Lungs, bronchial tubes, pleura, chest, breast.	Bronchitis, pleurisy, pneumonia, congestion, influenza.
4T	Gall bladder, common duct.	Gall bladder conditions, jaundice, shingles.
5T	Liver, solar plexus, blood.	Liver conditions, fevers, low blood pressure, anemia, poor circulation, arthritis.
6T	Stomach.	Stomach troubles, including nervous stomach, indigestion, heartburn, dyspepsia.
7T	Pancreas, duodenum.	Ulcers, gastritis.
8T	Spleen.	Lowered resistance.
9T	Adrenal and supra-renal glands.	Allergies, hives.
10T	Kidneys.	Kidney troubles, hardening of the arteries, chronic tiredness, nephritis, pyelitis.
11T	Kidneys, ureters.	Skin conditions such as acne, pimples, eczema, or boils.
12T	Small intestines, lymph circulation.	Rheumatism, gas pains, certain types of sterility.
1L	Large intestines, inguinal rings.	Constipation, colitis, dysentery, diarrhea, some ruptures or hernias.
2L	Appendix, abdomen, upper leg.	Cramps, difficult breathing, acidosis, varicose veins.
3L	Sex organs, uterus, bladder, knees.	Bladder troubles, menstrual troubles such as painful or irregular periods, miscarriages, bed wetting, impotency, change of life symptoms, many knee pains.
4L	Prostate gland, muscles of the lower back, sciatic nerve.	Sciatica; lumbago; difficult, painful, or too frequent urination; backaches.
5L	Lower legs, ankles, feet.	Poor circulation in the legs, swollen ankles, weak ankles and arches, cold feet, weakness in the legs, leg cramps.
SACRUM	Hip bones, buttocks.	Sacro-iliac conditions, spinal curvatures.
COCCYX	Rectum, anus.	Hemorrhoids (piles), pruritis (itching), pain at end of spine on sitting.

Some chiropractors use charts to promote the idea that spinal problems are a major cause of disease. This chart relates "spinal misalignments" and "irritation of the nervous system" to more than a hundred conditions, including allergies, amnesia, crossed eyes, deafness, hernias, kidney trouble, pneumonia, and thyroid problems. Some of the nerves do not actually go to the listed areas. Other charts showing how nerves run from the spine to the body's organs are used to persuade patients that regular spinal care is necessary for good health. This particular one was widely used during the 1970s and 1980s. Today's "nerve charts" tend to be more vaguely worded.

This "nerve chart" was included in a pamphlet for new patients published in 1975 by the Parker Chiropractic Research Foundation. The accompanying text stated: "Every cell of your body receives nerve impulses either directly or indirectly from the spine.... Locate the organ that is giving you the discomfort. Trace the nerve from the organ back to the spine. This nerve is the lifeline of the organ. If no nerve impulses reach the organ, it dies. If limited, or even increased, amount of impulses reaches it, the organ becomes sick. Normalize the nerve supply by a chiropractic adjustment, and normal function returns to the organ." The pamphlet was marketed until at least 1987, but a copy of the chart was included in a "Personal Chiropractic Report" that a chiropractor gave in 1998 to a patient I later treated.

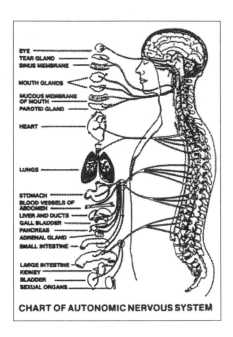

CHART OF AUTONOMIC NERVOUS SYSTEM

Overselling Spinal Adjustments

While tight joints can often be released with one or two manipulations, many chiropractors advise patients to undergo large numbers of spinal adjustments in order to correct their "subluxations" and prevent recurrence. Chiropractors who treat the "subluxation complex" often try to schedule treatments in advance, with frequent visits during the first few months, and gradually decreasing frequency until the patient is seen monthly—often for life—for what chiropractors call "preventative maintenance." Chapter 8 discusses this in more detail.

During 1989, William M. London, Ed.D., an assistant professor of health education at Kent State University, visited twenty-three chiropractors in Ohio and Florida who had advertised free consultations or examinations. All espoused subluxation theory either during the consultation or in waiting-room literature, and all but two recommended "preventative maintenance." In many cases, it is difficult to judge whether the chiropractor really believes multiple visits are necessary or whether they are simply a practice-building gimmick. Regardless, there is no scientific evidence that people who feel well should undergo periodic spinal checkups or adjustments.

Diagnostic Variations

Is it possible to diagnose a condition so nebulous that it cannot be clearly defined? The majority of chiropractors apparently think so—although they differ about how to do it. Some chiropractors—"straights" more so than "mixers"—believe subluxations are clearly visible on x-ray films. Some equivocate and say that x-ray evidence must be considered together with their clinical findings. Some practitioners x-ray the entire spine, while others use segmental films. Some utilize an x-ray marking system; others do not. "Super-straight" chiropractors typically describe what they do as "analysis" rather than "diagnosis" [74].

Some chiropractors find subluxations with one or another method of feeling along the spine with their hands. Other approaches include leg-length testing, weighing on twin scales, measuring skin temperature near the spine, measuring electrical activity of the muscles surrounding the spine, and interpreting patterns of light beamed onto the body surface. Chapter 10 discusses these various practices in detail. The main thing they have in common is lack of scientific validation.

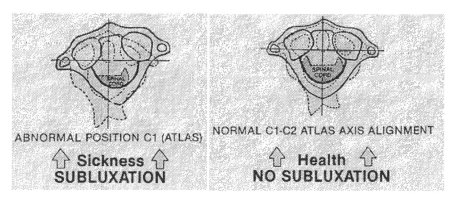

ABNORMAL POSITION C1 (ATLAS)   NORMAL C1-C2 ATLAS AXIS ALIGNMENT

⇧ **Sickness** ⇧   ⇧ **Health** ⇧
SUBLUXATION   **NO SUBLUXATION**

These images from a prominent "straight" chiropractor's Web site depict his conception of the top two vertebrae in health and disease. He states: "The 'Specific Chiropractor' ('Brain Stem Specialist') is trained to locate and remove this subluxation (misalignment) and restore the vertebrae to its normal position. The mental impulse life force, Innate Intelligence, can flow in its full capacity from the 'Brain Stem' to its diseased tissue or organ; healing or repair takes place in a natural way and pain and the ravenges [sic] of disease disappear." The site hosts an "International Directory of Brain Stem Specialists" and states: "The patients in these countries as well as in the US had positive results and some had complete recovery from such problems as Parkinson's Disease, AIDS, Paralysis, Sight and Hearing disorders" [98].

Treatment Variations

Chiropractic beliefs about treatment are as discordant as those about subluxations. More than a hundred "adjustive" techniques have been devised. Some chiropractors claim that specific vertebral levels correspond to specific organ dysfunctions and/or health problems (see charts on pages 6, 41, and 42). Some assert that the entire range of problems—including low-back pain—can be treated by manipulating only the neck. Some, as illustrated on page 43, focus only on the topmost vertebra (atlas). Some claim that only the lowermost vertebra (sacrum) needs attention. Some adjust both the atlas and the sacrum. Some adjust the entire spine in a shotgun approach. Chapter 11 discusses these approaches further. The main thing they have in common is lack of scientific testing.

Most of these approaches have several subvariations. Some practitioners "adjust" by hand; some use a small handheld device; and others use elaborate equipment. Manual adjustments can be delivered in many different ways. The most sensible chiropractors treat only the segments near areas of pain, restricted motion, or muscle spasm.

Physiologic Effects of Spinal Manipulation

While there is no reason to believe that a slight vertebral misalignment or any other spinal joint problem can "compromise neural integrity and influence organ system function and general health," spinal manipulation does have some physiologic effects on the body. It is well known, for example, that spinal manipulation, acupuncture, massage, and other forms of physical treatment can stimulate the body's production of endorphins to relieve pain. And like massage and other forms of stimulation applied to the body, including trauma, spinal manipulation can affect the activity of blood cells, increasing the defensive activity of white cells.

Immunological responses have been noted in the increased respiration of white cells following spinal manipulation [31]. It seems likely that similar responses could occur with any equivalent somatic treatment, including the stimulation of massage or hydrotherapy. But there is no reason to believe that any somatic therapy will cure any organic disease [127].

Regardless, none of the reactions resulting from somatic stimulation can be attributed to removing nerve interference caused by a misaligned vertebra. There is no reason at all to believe that a slightly misaligned vertebra, or a "subluxation complex," will have any effect at all on a spinal nerve or on muscle, connective, or vascular tissues. Contrary to the contentions of most chiropractors, the nervous system does not control all bodily functions. As noted by Scott Haldeman, M.D., Ph.D., D.C., a neurologist and third-generation chiropractor who teaches at the University of California, "There are very strong chemical and hormonal control systems, very strong local homeostatic systems, very strong vascular control systems. To emphasize one system over another is a position of bias" [37].

"Curing" Simulated Disease

Manipulation sometimes produces dramatic relief of symptoms that mimic those of a visceral disease. Pain can be referred to most parts of the body by an irritated spinal nerve. For example, an irritated thoracic spinal nerve can produce pain in the chest or arm that resembles angina pectoris. The disappearance of such a pain following spinal manipulation might be misinterpreted as a cure for heart disease.

While spinal problems can refer pain into musculoskeletal structures to simulate visceral disease, and visceral problems can refer pain into musculoskeletal structures, there is no reason to believe that pinching or irritation of a spinal nerve will have an adverse effect on visceral function. The body's organs are largely under the control of the autonomic nervous system, which is not affected by injury to a spinal nerve. Severing the spinal cord can result in paralysis in musculoskeletal structures without loss of visceral function. There are, however, fibers connecting the autonomic nervous system with spinal nerves so that musculoskeletal structures receive such autonomic functions as sensation or sweating over skin surface. Because of these connector fibers, a heart muscle pain may be referred back through spinal nerves to the chest and left arm. But pinching spinal nerves that supply the left arm would not adversely affect the heart.

Disk herniation or a bony spur can pinch or irritate a spinal nerve at the intervertebral foramen, but impaired spinal nerves have never been demonstrated to affect body organs, much less general health. If slight vertebral misalignments could pinch spinal nerves or damage people's health, the human race would not have survived.

Summing It Up

Subluxation theory, less influential than it was decades ago, remains deeply rooted within the chiropractic profession. However, I would be remiss if this chapter left you with the impression that all chiropractors are muddleheads or that everything they do is wrong. Rational chiropractors—even some that espouse subluxation theories—can do a lot to help people with back trouble or other musculoskeletal conditions. The vast majority of those who consult chiropractors are seeking pain relief, and most are satisfied with their results. This book's purpose is to help consumers procure the benefits while avoiding the pitfalls. It dwells on the negative because—quite frankly—so much of chiropractic is problematic. To safely navigate the chiropractic marketplace, it is necessary to be well informed.

Rational chiropractors *do* exist, and—particularly in recent years—their number is increasing. Most clear-thinking chiropractors work unobtrusively in their offices, as did I and my father before me. Chiropractic education—particularly at the more medically oriented chiropractic colleges—has improved greatly. And serious research is being done to try to figure out what chiropractors are doing correctly.

The next chapter traces the history of chiropractic education, including the extent to which subluxation theory is taught in the schools.

5

How Good Is Chiropractic Education?

Do chiropractic schools prepare their graduates to properly care for patients? In 1968, a comprehensive study by the U.S. Department of Health, Education, and Welfare concluded they did not:

> Chiropractic theory and practice are not based upon the body of knowledge related to health, disease, and health care that has been widely accepted by the scientific community. Moreover, irrespective of its theory, the scope and quality of chiropractic education do not prepare the practitioner to make an adequate diagnosis and provide adequate treatment. [42]

Although chiropractic schools have improved considerably since that time, most still teach subluxation theory, and some still instruct students to treat "subluxations" rather than diseases or "conditions." Before focusing on the current situation, let's briefly review the checkered history of chiropractic education.

Serious Shortcomings

The total number of chiropractic schools that have existed is unknown. A scholarly review has located evidence of about 400, of which 188 had a traceable record of existence for longer than a year [58]. In 1980, chiropractic historian Russell W. Gibbons categorized chiropractic's educational development into four periods of activity:

1. The Tutorial Period (1897–1905), during which D.D. Palmer conveyed his ideas to his earliest followers. During this period, the course grew from three weeks to three months.
2. The Classical Period (1905–1924), during which chiropractic emerged from an informal curriculum to established didactic and clinical experiences.
3. The Proprietary Period (1924–1960), during which there was much internal debate about educational reform and groundwork was laid for standardization and accreditation.
4. The Professional Period (1960–1980), during which schools consolidated, campuses were renovated, and teaching facilities were upgraded [67].

The earliest chiropractic diplomas stated that the holder was competent to teach as well as to practice, a situation that encouraged graduates to open their own schools. Between 1906 and 1924, the number of schools increased to at least sixty-four and the length of instruction at the Palmer School of Chiropractic was raised from three months to eighteen months [142:341]. However, the quality of these schools was extremely low. As noted by Morris Fishbein, M.D.:

> When Dr. Thomas F. Duhigg reported the results of an inspection of the schools in Davenport for the Pennsylvania Bureau of Medical Education and Licensure, he pointed out that in 1915 the three colleges which had developed in that capitol of chiropractic were really little fit to educate anybody in anything. None had a library, a hospital, a laboratory worthy of the name, post-mortems [autopsies], or capable teachers. To these institutions came students without preliminary education, and after one year of study in miserably equipped buildings, consisting mostly of lecture halls and demonstration rooms, they were turned loose to minister to the sick. . . .
>   When Dr. George Dock visited the fountainhead of chiropractic in 1921 . . . Palmer's original plant had expanded into a series of buildings. . . . But the large buildings, Dock reported, were still not devoted to teaching any of the fundamental facts of physiology, pathology, bacteriology, or even hygiene or sanitation. [60]

Although the Palmer School relied on standard medical textbooks for some of its teachings, it did not use them as their authors would have intended. As recently noted in the journal of the History of Science Society:

> Lecture notes from the early years . . .provide an excellent example of how chiropractors transformed the meaning of facts widely

accepted by orthodox scientists. Prior to the development of a series of chiropractic texts that covered basic science subjects such as anatomy and physiology, the Palmer School used standard medical textbooks. B.J. Palmer's lecture notes for these courses specified which sections of the medical works students should read. When the texts contained materials antithetical to the chiropractic approach or ignored facts integral to it—for example, the importance of Innate Intelligence—the lecture notes directed the student to delete or modify these passages so as to offer appropriate chiropractic information. [122]

In the late 1950s, the Stanford Research Institute (SRI) evaluated three Los Angeles schools that had produced 71 percent of the chiropractors practicing within California. One of the schools would not permit inspection. SRI's 254-page report, issued in 1960, was extremely negative. Among its conclusions:

> Chiropractic schools use course titles and textbooks similar to those used in medical and osteopathic schools. However, their teaching approach is centered almost entirely on classroom lectures and practical work in outpatient clinics. No hospital inpatient training is available.
>
> Although a number of laboratory courses are listed in school catalogues, there was no evidence that the chemistry laboratories were in use at any time during Institute project team visits. . . . Similarly, the libraries were found to be seldom used. . . . Circulation records, accession lists, and certain other controls used in libraries were not established. The laboratories were not equipped and the libraries were not staffed to serve the purposes for which they were intended. These conditions suggest that libraries and laboratories do not play an important role in the education of a chiropractor. [182]

In 1963, the Canadian College of Physicians and Surgeons of the Province of Quebec published a lengthy report that concluded: "The education of chiropractors is unacceptable because in schools of chiropractic the numbers and training of the teachers, as well as the organization of the courses, are far below minimum standards."

That same year, the AMA Department of Investigation submitted an inquiry from a fictitious person to seven of the fifteen chiropractic colleges then operating. One letter stated that its eighteen-year-old writer didn't want to waste time at regular college because "everyone I ever knew who went to . . . colleges around here always flunked out" and that he wanted to "make a lot of money and still not have to go to school all your life like some doctors." The other six inquiries were equally inappropriate. Nevertheless, all seven schools sent application packets and five applicants were accepted even though none submitted evidence of a high school diploma or equivalency certificate that was supposedly required for admission [5].

The AMA Department of Investigation then evaluated the credentials of faculty members listed in the catalogs of the thirteen chiropractic colleges that had been approved by chiropractic accrediting agencies. Fewer than half had graduated from college, and many who taught basic sciences did not have any degree in the subjects they taught [6].

The 1968 HEW report's sections on chiropractic education and research concluded:

> Two notable features of the chiropractic educational system should be mentioned: first, the wide range of the courses, which indicates an effort, in principle at least, to give to students a basic knowledge similar to that of medicine and osteopathy; and second, efforts at self-improvement. . . .
>
> However, significant shortcomings in chiropractic education include: (1) Lack of inpatient hospital training; (2) Lack of adequately qualified faculty; (3) Extremely low admission requirements for students; (4) Lack of a nationally recognized accreditation body; (5) Such dissension within the profession that two separate accreditation programs must be maintained.
>
> These shortcomings raise serious doubts as to the qualifications of chiropractors generally to make an adequate diagnosis and effectively treat patients. The doubts are compounded when seen in the light of the chiropractic philosophy, which has been shown to deemphasize proven factors in the causation of disease and the necessity for differential diagnosis and for therapy other than manipulation. Thus, it appears doubtful that improvement in the educational program can proceed, despite efforts in that direction, until: (1) The need for differential diagnosis and forms of therapy other than manipulation is recognized; (2) Fully qualified, specialized faculty are available to teach the scientific courses.
>
> Some difficulties are encountered by nonchiropractors in evaluating chiropractic research. One is that the nonchiropractor looks for documentation of diagnosis, the accuracy of which is central to the validity of the research; but to the chiropractor, naming the disease is not so important . . . since subluxation is considered the cause of the illness. This raises the problem of definitions, since the nonchiropractor may not understand the chiropractor's interpretation of this causal relationship. Measurements of "improvement" also present problems, the nonchiropractor looking for specific

indices to show improvement. In one chiropractic study, improvement is shown in terms of readings on a "neurocalograph," an instrument that is not used for this purpose in other disciplines. Finally, tests of statistical significance are difficult to apply to chiropractic research, due to small study samples. [42]

Efforts at Reform

Until the mid-1930s, chiropractic was taught only in private schools. The National Chiropractic Association (NCA) formed a Committee on Educational Standards (CES) in 1935 and an accrediting agency called the Council on Chiropractic Education (CCE) in 1947. By 1948, because of pressure from a CES official, many NCA-affiliated schools had closed and the rest had merged into eight nonprofit institutions [182]. In 1963, the NCA became the American Chiropractic Association. CCE became autonomous in 1971 and was recognized by the U.S. Office of Education (USOE) in 1974. Following this, state laws were gradually amended to require new applicants to possess a chiropractic degree from a school accredited by a recognized accrediting agency. These laws made it increasingly difficult and eventually impossible for nonaccredited schools to attract students.

During the 1950s, after the NCA developed standards for "mixer" colleges, the International Chiropractors Association published accreditation standards for the remaining "straight" schools. However, it eventually became a CCE cosponsor, and some of the schools it accredited obtained CCE approval. In 1978, three "straight" colleges formed a third agency, the Straight Chiropractic Academic Standards Association (SCASA), which received USOE approval in 1988 but lost it in 1993. One school modified its curriculum and became CCE-accredited in 1995, but the others closed [185].

Today, admission to a CCE-accredited school requires two years of prechiropractic college education with at least a C average. To receive the doctor of chiropractic (D.C.) degree, students must complete a minimum of 4,200 hours of study over a four-year period. The courses include anatomy, biochemistry, microbiology, pathology, physiology, public health, obstetrics, pediatrics, geriatrics, dermatology, otolaryngology, diagnostic imaging procedures, psychology, nutrition/dietetics, biomechanics, orthopedics, first aid and emergency procedures, chiropractic principles and practice, adjustive techniques, research methods, and professional ethics [50].

CCE sets standards for the curriculum, faculty and staff, facilities, patient care, and research. Accreditation is awarded periodically for up to seven years at a time. Each school is required to set its own goals and to assess its strengths, weaknesses, and educational outcomes. During each cycle, a CCE team of educators and practitioners visits to review compliance with CCE standards and the institution's mission and goals [36:18]. However, none of this ensures that the teachings are valid or on a par with medical educational standards. The entire process is contaminated by CCE's willingness to tolerate the teaching of subluxation dogma. Chiropractic reform efforts might be enhanced if USOE had higher standards. Scientific validity is not among its criteria for approving accrediting agencies for training health-care practitioners! [120:50]

Chiropractic versus Medical Education

Chiropractors often suggest that their schooling is similar or equivalent to that of medical doctors, except that chiropractic schools emphasize the management of musculoskeletal disorders rather than treatment with drugs and surgery. This description is overly optimistic. As Dr. Stephen Barrett has noted:

> Chiropractic schools do not provide the depth of diagnostic and therapeutic training that physicians receive. Whereas most medical school faculties are large and contain experts in every aspect of medical practice, chiropractic schools have few or no physicians on their faculty. While the patients studied by medical students encompass the full range of disease, the vast majority seen by chiropractic students seek help for musculoskeletal problems. Although some of their courses are based on standard medical textbooks, chiropractic students lack the experiences needed to make the information meaningful. Chiropractic instruction in such subjects as pediatrics, obstetrics, and gynecology is usually limited to the classroom, with little or no actual patient contact and no experience with hospitalized patients. Life College, for example, uses only rubber models to teach students how to perform pelvic and rectal examinations. Critics charge that because much of chiropractic is based on a false premise, neither length of study nor accreditation of its schools can ensure that those who graduate will practice competently. [23]

Many chiropractic schools require their students to recruit patients in order to meet minimum clinical requirements for graduation (see box on CCE accreditation criteria). This was brought to public attention in a recent lawsuit by Julie Burnet, a former student who charged that Cleveland Chiropractic College had committed fraud by failing to tell her that she would be responsible for recruiting her own patients during the clinical phase of chiropractic training. Burnet testified that to meet quotas, students were required to lure or entice friends and family into the clinic, and then charge them for chiropractic treatment that they did not need. A former instructor testified that between 1991 and 1995, she knew of no student who met the clinical requirements solely by relying on patients provided by the clinic. In 1996, a jury awarded $93,000 in actual damages plus $45,000 in punitive damages [124].

Another reflection of educational quality is admission standards. A recent study found that chiropractic school standards were lower than those

---

CCE Criteria for Accreditation (Excerpt)

The program or institution must provide evidence that demonstrates that the degree candidates, as a condition of graduation, have:

(a) performed at least twenty-five (25) clinical examinations with case history for the purpose of developing a diagnostic or clinical impression of the status of the patient relative to chiropractic care.

(b) perform and interpret, order and interpret, or interpret at least twenty-five (25) area radiographic (diagnostic imaging) examinations with written reports of findings.

(c) interpreted clinical laboratory tests to include at least twenty-five (25) urinalyses, twenty (20) hematology procedures such as complete blood counts, and ten (10) clinical chemistry, microbiology or immunology procedures or profiles on human blood and/or other body fluids.

(d) performed a minimum of 80% chiropractic spinal adjustments and/or manipulations during at least 250 separate patient care visits.

(e) integrated the elements of the basic, chiropractic, clinical sciences and clinical instruction into clinical decisions.

No more than twenty (20) percent of appropriate services may be administered to students and/or student's families.

The degree candidate must have ordered, performed, and integrated the data for case management and follow-up from appropriate services of those listed above on a minimum of ten (10) different outpatients as a requirement for graduation.

From: *Standards for Chiropractic Programs and Institutions Council on Chiropractic Education*, January 1995 [50].

Table 5-1. Characteristics of Students Entering Professional Schools

Type and Number of Schools	% Bachelor's Degree	Avg. Minimum GPA Required	Avg. GPA of Enrollees
Medical (17)	99.35%	3.16	3.56
Optometry (16)	76.88%	2.55	3.30
Osteopathic (16	97.00%	2.68	3.26
Dental (15)	66.87%	2.79	3.13
Podiatry (7)	89.40%	2.76	3.06
Chiropractic (16)	42.25%	2.38	2.90

Source: Doxey TT, Phillips RB. Comparison of entrance requirements for health care professions. JMPT 20:86–91, 1997.

at five other types of professional schools (see table above). The researchers tabulated the percentage of the previous year's entering class with a bachelor's degree, the minimum grade point average (GPA) required for admission, and the average GPA of the previous year's enrollees. They noted that although undergraduate success may reflect the potential for professional success, further research would be needed to confirm this [55].

Unlike chiropractic, which is guided by a doctrine that permits an unlimited practice with a limited treatment method, science-based medicine is unlimited in both scope of practice and treatment methods and is free to adopt any treatment method of value. Physicians who use drugs and surgery and who must handle medical emergencies obviously need more education than a chiropractor who does none of these things. But both should be equally competent in making a diagnosis. Chiropractic fails to place proper limitations upon practitioners whose diagnostic abilities and treatment methods are not adequate for the scope of practice they claim.

Medical schools require four years of training, but nearly everyone who graduates takes at least three more additional years of specialty training. While chiropractic education may be adequate for treating mechanical-type musculoskeletal problems, critics question how well it prepares students to diagnose the conditions under which spinal manipulation should *not* be done [129]. Remember, too, that subluxation theory minimizes the importance of diagnosis. Some "straight" chiropractors maintain that they do not diagnose and treat disease but merely adjust subluxations so the body can heal itself.

The Subluxation Spectrum

Some chiropractic colleges are more fundamentalistic than others, with some teaching "straight" or pure chiropractic and others teaching "mixed" chiropractic or concentrating more upon the care of musculoskeletal conditions. Nearly all describe chiropractic as a method of correcting subluxations or improving the relationship between structure and function in the spine. To my knowledge, all chiropractic colleges teach that spinal adjustments can improve health. In fact, the Association of Chiropractic Colleges, a consortium that includes all of the American chiropractic schools plus one in Canada, has issued a position paper—excerpted on the following page—stating that "the purpose of chiropractic is to optimize health" [13].

In 1993, when there were eighteen chiropractic colleges in the United States, *The Chiropractic Journal* (a newspaper that advocates "straight" philosophy) sent each of their presidents a letter asking whether his school taught students how to locate and correct vertebral subluxations and that subluxation correction is the foundation for their practice. All fourteen who answered either said "yes" or indicated that the topic was an integral part of their curriculum. Three of the "straight" college presidents even said that their students were taught to treat subluxations rather than diseases or "conditions" [196]. The presidents of the three most scientifically oriented schools—Los Angeles College of Chiropractic, National College of Chiropractic, and Western States Chiropractic College—chose not to answer. Recent literature packets from these schools do not mention the "s" word, but they still imply—ambiguously—that spinal problems are a factor in ill health and that chiropractic care may help a broad spectrum of problems. The 1997–1999 Los Angeles catalog, for example, states:

> The teaching of chiropractic treatment at LACC for both neuro-musculoskeletal and non-neuromusculoskeletal conditions is based on scientific principles and sound hypotheses. . . . Chiropractic care is directed toward the restoration of health primarily influencing the nervous system by adjustments of the spine and other joints of the body. [119]

National College has a vigorous research department and publishes two of chiropractic's scientific journals, the *Journal of Manipulative and Physiological Therapeutics* (JMPT) and *Chiropractic Technique*. A 1998 fact sheet states that "chiropractic is not and does not profess to be an all-inclusive art of healing. It acknowledges limitations, recognizes the need for consultation and referral, and is respectfully aware of the efficacy of

**Position Paper on Chiropractic and Subluxation
Association of Chiropractic Colleges (Excerpts, 1996)**

Chiropractic is a health care discipline which emphasizes the inherent recuperative power of the body to heal itself without the use of drugs or surgery. The practice of chiropractic focuses on the relationship between structure (primarily the spine) and function (as coordinated by the nervous system) and how that relationship affects the preservation and restoration of health. In addition, Doctors of Chiropractic recognize the value and responsibility of working in cooperation with other health care practitioners when in the best interest of the patient. . . .

The purpose of chiropractic is to optimize health. The body's innate recuperative power is affected by and integrated through the nervous system.

The practice of chiropractic includes: establishing a diagnosis; facilitating neurological and biomechanical integrity through appropriate chiropractic case management; and promoting health. The foundation of chiropractic includes philosophy, science, art, knowledge, and clinical experience. . . .

Chiropractic is concerned with the preservation and restoration of health, and focuses particular attention on the subluxation. A subluxation is a complex of functional and/or structural and/or pathological articular changes that compromise neural integrity and may influence organ system function and general health. A subluxation is evaluated, diagnosed, and managed through the use of chiropractic procedures based on the best available rational and empirical evidence. [13]

Source: ACC Web site, December 1998.

other forms of therapy." Yet the document also implies that chiropractic's scope may be unlimited:

> The basic distinguishing principle underlying the practice of chiropractic, differentiating it from the other healing arts and sciences, is the fact that disturbances of the nervous system produced by derangements within the spine and pelvis are often a primary or contributing factor in the pathological process of many common or seemingly intractable human ailments. [57]

Western States has a unique program aimed at integrating chiropractors into the medical mainstream. It recently added several medical doctors to its faculty, added classes in relevant drug treatment to its curriculum, and announced that it will award a Doctor of Chiropractic Medicine (D.C.M.)

degree. It openly teaches that immunizations are useful and has held vaccination clinics on its campus. Since it is a chiropractic college, Western States teaches courses in chiropractic philosophy, principles, and adjustive techniques. But the college's emphasis on neuromusculoskeletal problems, with appropriate use of drug therapy in combination with conservative treatment methods that include use of spinal manipulation, offers promise for more integrated, complete care for back pain and other musculoskeletal problems in a chiropractic setting. Needless to say, many chiropractors and "straight" chiropractic educators have denounced the "medicalization" of Western States.

Sherman College of Straight Chiropractic lies at the other end of the subluxation spectrum. It teaches that subluxations are the primary cause of disease and that a chiropractor's true role is not to treat disease, but to locate, analyze, and correct subluxations. "Today," according to a 1998 issue of Sherman's *Bulletin,* "Chiropractic has evolved into a highly developed science and art which deals not with disease, but with vertebral subluxation and its effect on the body's natural striving toward health" [167]. Making a special effort to distinguish itself from other chiropractic schools, the college defines its mission this way:

> There exists, within the chiropractic profession today, two schools of thought.
> "Straight" chiropractic uses chiropractic methods of examination, analysis, and adjusting to accomplish the objective of correcting vertebral subluxation. Vertebral subluxation is a condition in which a vertebra becomes slightly misaligned with an adjacent segment in such a way as to disturb nerve function, interfering with the body's striving to maintain its own health.
> The other school of thought, "mixer" chiropractic, uses manipulation (similar to adjustments) and other methods which accomplish the objective of treating symptoms and disease.
> "Straight" means a total commitment to the teaching, research and practice of chiropractic focused on correcting vertebral subluxation. The word "straight" is in the College's name to identify it with this distinct mission. [167]

Although Palmer College's catalog does not openly disparage diagnosis, it clearly reflects the beliefs of its founders.

> Chiropractic employs neither drugs nor surgery. It is concerned with the entire environment of the body and is based on a properly functioning nervous system, which begins with the brain and courses through the spinal cord encased within the spinal column. No part of the body escapes the dominance of the nervous system.

Spinal biomechanical dysfunction—improper joint function at a specific point in the spine due to slight misalignments called subluxations—may cause a state of poor health in an area far removed from the spine and spinal cord itself. The lightest pressure by a vertebra may alter the regular transmission of nerve impulses, preventing that portion of the body from responding with its full inherent capacity to demands for proper function.

A chiropractic adjustment (the application of a precise force to a specific part of the spinal segment), corrects the vertebral subluxation, permitting normal nerve transmission and recuperative capability. [139]

Life College, the largest of the chiropractic schools, is equally imbued with subluxation dogma. Its 1997 catalog states:

The School of Chiropractic of Life College seeks to instill within its students the non-duplicating principles set forth by D.D. Palmer, his son, B.J. Palmer, and other dedicated pioneers who have helped to develop Chiropractic as a science, i.e., the relationship between structure, primarily the spine, and function primarily coordinated by the nervous system of the human body as that relationship may affect the restoration and preservation of health without use of drugs and/or surgery. [116]

Life's founder and president, Sid Williams, D.C., is probably the profession's most evangelistic leader. In a recent article, he stated: "I have never found any justification for doing anything for, or to, a patient who comes to me for chiropractic care, other than doing the best job possible of adjusting that patient's spine" [200]. In a report posted to the Chirobase Web site, Allen J. Botnick, D.C., a 1996 Life graduate, has vividly described Williams's teachings at the school's assemblies, which all students and faculty are required to attend [29]. (See box on next page.)

A school's printed curriculum doesn't tell the whole story, however. At least four other factors help determine what students believe and do after they graduate. First, many students have firm subluxation-based beliefs before they begin school. Many are either children of a chiropractor or have been raised in an atmosphere of chiropractic belief (including weekly or monthly spinal adjustments). Such students may not only graduate with dogmatic beliefs, but may also exert pressure on their classmates. (At some schools, nonbelievers are openly ridiculed.) Second, faculty members have a wide spectrum of beliefs, even at the more progressive schools. Third, invalid procedures are promoted through student clubs and by visiting lecturers. Fourth, practicing chiropractors are flooded with solicitations to

Some Notes on Life College's Assembly and Its Money Hum
Allen J. Botnick, D.C.

Sid Williams believes that chiropractors should be the primary-health care providers to the nation. He agreed with B.J. Palmer that manipulation would empty the asylums, prisons, and hospitals. He said that by releasing the innate vital force, natural immunity would be raised, restoring homeostasis. The reason chiropractic had not yet become widely utilized for health, we were told, was because of a medical conspiracy. He stated that eventually medical doctors who believed in the germ theory would all commit suicide when they realized that the most important factor to health was homeostasis. Nearly all the students appeared to accept his teaching that manipulations were not just for back pain but were a necessary part of maintaining health.

Sid used some of his time to teach us tricks of the trade. He told us personal stories, like how he took a job as a traveling salesperson selling aluminum pots and pans to pay for chiropractic college. He said he didn't become successful until he started believing in his products. We were told to lavish love on our patients with firm handshakes and by saying "Glad ta see ya." We were advised on how to use leading questions to plant uncertainty into a person's mind, hopefully recruiting them and their family as patients. This was condoned because we were saving them from "killer subluxations" that they didn't even know they had.

Sid told us that meditation and visualization were powerful. Many times he led us in a meditation or demonstrated a breathing exercise. The most notable was the "Money Hum," which he said was designed to help us achieve fabulous success as chiropractors by getting over our school-induced poverty consciousness. Sid said that the reason people fail in practice was not due to tangible reasons like excessive student loans or lack of business experience, but to a bad mindset and lack of belief in the chiropractic "Big Idea" that everyone needs an adjustment. Sid instructed us:

> Stand up everyone. Close your eyes and bend your knees to get low to the ground. Now I want you to start humming. MMMMMMMMMMMMM. Visualize piles and piles of dollar bills up to your chin. Visualize a line of patients outside the door of your clinic waiting to be adjusted. You can almost feel the money, touch it. Now, grab a big handful and thrust your hand up in a fist towards the sky while saying MMMMMONEY!!

The exercise would be repeated three times to be sure everyone got it right.

Sid's other big topic was criticizing medically oriented chiropractic schools and doctors. He opposed chiropractors using any treatments other than manipulation. He joked about it in assembly, but the school actually outlawed the use of all methods of treatment it deemed medically oriented in both the student and outpatient clinics. [29]

attend seminars on subluxation-based practice-building techniques, invalid diagnostic approaches, unsubstantiated nutrition treatments, and other dubious practices. To my knowledge, no chiropractic school, mainstream chiropractic organization, or chiropractic publication has ever made a determined effort to discourage these dubious beliefs and practices.

Although it is possible to graduate from a straight school without any belief in subluxation theory, the percentage of students doing so is probably small. The situation has been aptly summarized by Joseph C. Keating, Jr., Ph.D., a research expert who currently teaches at Los Angeles Chiropractic College:

> Several of the largest and some of the smallest student bodies in the profession today are found at institutions that emphasize biotheology, vitalism, pseudo-science, and marketing values. . . . Most in the profession are aware of where the "phooolosophical" leaders in chiropractic education reside. These schools are busy turning out "brand new, old-fashioned chiropractors," investigating Innate . . . and "proving" what they always knew was true. . . . And although many graduates of these theological institutions can be expected to reject the most absurd ideas promoted by their presidents and boards, . . . we are faced nonetheless with the alarming reality that a whole new generation of (well meaning) dingbat doctors . . . advertising fanatics, and evangelical ideologists will be with us for many years to come. [102]

The Bottom Line

Although chiropractic educational requirements have steadily increased, these advances have had little influence on chiropractic dogma. With few exceptions, chiropractic colleges still teach subluxation theory and permit philosophy to overshadow science. While some students acquire sufficient skill to manage various musculoskeletal problems, others emerge with an affinity for nonsense. The next several chapters describe this problem in detail.

6

The ABCs
of Back Pain

Low-back pain is a widespread problem. From 60 to 80 percent of adults will have it during their lifetime, and 2 to 5 percent will have it at any given time. In the United States, it is the fifth most common problem for which people visit a medical or osteopathic physician [204] and the most common reason why people consult chiropractors [88]. The total direct and indirect costs attributable to back pain in the United States are estimated to run as high as $60 billion per year [164]. Although its symptoms are usually acute and self-limiting, low-back pain often recurs and, in 5 to 10 percent of patients, it becomes chronic.

What should you do if you get a backache? How can you judge its seriousness? When should you seek professional help? Should you see a medical doctor or a chiropractor? To answer these questions, it helps to know something about the anatomy of the back.

Basic Concepts

The structures of the back include the spinal bones (vertebrae), their joints (facet joints), the disks between the vertebrae, and the muscles and ligaments that hold these structures together. The backbone supports the body's weight. The facet joints enable the spine to twist and bend. The intervertebral disks serve as shock absorbers. The vertebrae help protect the spinal cord from injury. Openings in each vertebra line up to form a long hollow canal through which the spinal cord runs downward from the base of the brain to the second lumbar vertebra (L2). Along the way it gives off branches (nerve roots) that serve all the muscles and skin except for those of the head. At approximately L2, the cord forms many branches that exit through openings in the lower lumbar and sacral portions of the spine. The branches resemble the hair hanging down from a horse's tail, the Latin term for which is *cauda equina.*

Any of these structures can be injured. Ligaments and muscles can be sprained or strained by a sudden or improper movement, or by overuse. (A sprain is a stretch or tear of a ligament; a strain is a stretching injury of a muscle.) Disks can become similarly damaged so that they bulge or tear. If a tear is large enough, gelatinous material can leak out and press against a spinal nerve, a condition referred to as a herniated or "ruptured" disk. Pain caused by muscular strain is usually confined to the back, is accompanied by stiffness, and typically occurs during movements such as bending or twisting. Minor cases usually resolve within a few days. Back pain that is severe, radiates into the calf or foot, and is accompanied by numbness or tingling, may be a sign of nerve-root compression caused by disk herniation. Spinal nerves can also become swollen or inflamed for other reasons. Pain originating in the lumbar area and radiating down back of the leg along the distribution of the sciatic nerve (see figure below) is called sciatic pain or sciatica.

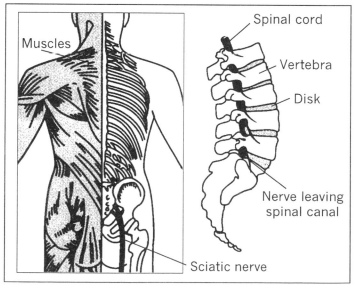

Structures of the back and spine.

Acute back pain is defined as back pain or back-related leg pain severe enough to restrict activity less than three months. About 90 percent of patients with acute low-back pain spontaneously recover activity tolerance within one month. Severe pain caused by a muscle spasm usually lasts two or three days and is followed by gradual healing and pain reduction. If the affected area is not reinjured, recovery should be complete within eight to twelve weeks.

Back pain can also be caused by problems of the bones and joints. Arthritis pain is usually a steady ache. Compression fractures produce sudden pain, often without an apparent reason. Compression fractures in the middle or low back are usually the result of osteoporosis, a condition in which the bones become thinner and weaker. Less common causes of acute back pain include tumors, kidney problems, and pain referred from diseases of various other internal organs.

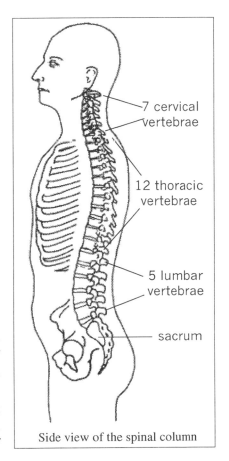

Side view of the spinal column

7 cervical vertebrae

12 thoracic vertebrae

5 lumbar vertebrae

sacrum

Self-Assessment

Most backaches result from simple mechanical-type strains that will resolve spontaneously within a few weeks. The causes include lifting a heavy object and lifting from an awkward position. If you develop back pain for the first time as the result of a simple strain or stumble, it may not be necessary to rush to a doctor's office. You won't need an x-ray examination unless the pain persists for several weeks or a fracture, infection, tumor, or neurological defect is suspected.

If you fall or hurt your back lifting something, or if you suddenly feel pain during an awkward movement, the mechanical origin of the pain will usually be obvious. Often, however, back pain occurs for no apparent reason and you may have difficulty deciding what problem you have and what type of doctor you should see.

Some preliminary tests can help you determine whether the problem is mechanical or is a sign of some disease. Pain on movement is usually a reliable sign that back pain has a mechanical cause. In typical cases, bending over, getting out of a chair, or turning over in bed will cause pain to occur in an injured or painful spinal segment. Unless the injury is severe, rest will usually ease the pain.

A pinched spinal nerve causing pain to radiate down one leg may interfere with forward movement of the leg. To test for sciatic nerve involvement, lie on your back with your legs straight. Then have another person lift the affected leg as far as possible with a hand cupped below your ankle and your leg completely limp. If there is a pinched nerve in the lower lumbar area of your spine, you may feel pain in your back and buttock on the side of the leg pain with less than 60 degrees of straight leg raising (SLR). This occurs because stretching the sciatic nerve causes pulling on the spinal nerve that is pinched. The most common cause is a herniated disk.

Severe pain accompanied by numbness or tingling in the affected thigh or leg is often a sign that a nerve is undergoing damage which, if uncorrected, will result in weakness and loss of sensation in the muscles and skin supplied by the affected nerve. Nerve-root encroachment in the lumbar spine causes symptoms that extend into the thigh or the lower leg. But the location of the symptoms depends upon which portion of the lumbar spine is involved. Symptoms of the thigh may result from nerve involvement of the second (L2) or the third (L3) lumbar nerves in the upper portion of the

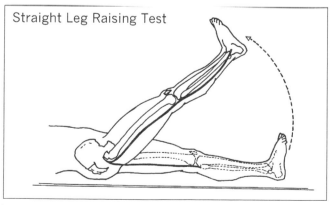

Straight Leg Raising Test

Pain that occurs when the sciatic nerve is stretched with less than 60 degrees of straight leg raising is a sign that a spinal nerve is being pinched.

lumbar spine. Symptoms in the lower leg may originate from nerve involvement in the lower lumbar spine. Damage to the fourth lumbar nerve (L4) might cause numbness on the inside of the lower leg, while damage to the fifth lumbar nerve might cause loss of sensation on the outside of the lower leg and on top of the foot. True sciatica involving L5 and S1 nerves is most often characterized by pain radiating from the back and buttock into the outside portion of the leg and foot.

More than 90 percent of lower back disk herniations occur in the lower lumbar region. This means that nerve problems originating in the lumbar spine most commonly cause symptoms that extend below the knee. Problems in the upper lumbar area can cause weakness in the thigh. Three simple tests can help determine whether you have nerve impingement or damage and where the problem might be located.

Heel walk: Try walking on your heels, keeping the forepart of both feet off the floor. If you are unable to keep one of your feet from dropping flat to the floor, you might have "foot drop," a sign of nerve damage caused by an L4 or L5 disk herniation.

Toe walk: Try walking on your toes, keeping the heels of both feet off the floor. If the heel of one foot falls to the floor and you are unable to walk on your toes, you might have nerve damage due to an L5 disk herniation. If you discover weakness of your foot or leg, you should see a doctor for further examination. The doctor will check your ankle reflexes, test the strength of your legs, measure your calves for muscle shrinkage, and test your skin for loss of sensitivity.

Squat Test: Hold on to a bedpost and squat halfway down, first favoring one leg and then the other. If one of your thighs is weak, you might have nerve damage that is the result of an upper lumbar disk herniation. The knee reflex can be tested by tapping just below the kneecap with the edge of a thin book. Weakness of a thigh muscle or absence of a knee reflex are reasons to consult a doctor.

Back pain caused by a kidney stone is usually severe. Unlike a mechanical-type problem that causes pain when you move, forcing you to remain as still as possible, the pain caused by a kidney stone will usually cause you to keep moving. Kidney pain, which typically radiates into the groin and the inside of the thigh on the side of the stone, is often accompanied by nausea and a cold sweat. If you suspect that you might have a kidney stone, contact your doctor to find out whether you should go to the office or to a hospital emergency room.

Table 6-1. When to Consult a Doctor for Back Pain

- Pain that is severe or worsens when lying down
- Unexplained fever over 100°F
- Pain that is present for more than a month without improvement, or occurs at rest, or is worsening
- Unexplained weight loss
- History of cancer
- Long-term steroid use, which can weaken the bones and increase susceptibility to fractures
- Recent onset of urinary tract problems, such as pain or burning on urination, increased frequency, or infection
- Trauma capable of causing a fracture, such as a high-impact auto accident or a serious fall
- In the elderly, minor trauma, especially if the person has osteoporosis
- Severe weakness or numbness in a leg, the genital area, or the buttocks; or change in the ability to urinate or have a bowel movement. These are signs of possible spinal nerve impairment.

Remember that sudden onset of back pain following a simple exertion or a fall (involving persons who are not elderly and who do not have a history of disease) is usually a simple strain. Incapacitating back pain caused by severe injury may be the result of a joint or ligament sprain, a herniated disk, or a spinal fracture. In such cases, you should consult an orthopedist before undergoing treatment with physical therapy or manipulation.

Table 6-1 summarizes the signs and symptoms indicating that a doctor should be consulted.

Visiting a Doctor

The first thing most doctors will do if you seek treatment for back pain is observe how you walk. If walking is difficult and movement is painful, it is likely that your problem is mechanical and not the result of an infection or an internal problem. Inspection of the bare back may reveal some tilting of the spine due to muscle spasm, which often pulls the body forward or to one side, restricting range of motion. Simple percussion, or jarring the spine with a closed fist, will often locate the painful segment if the pain originates in a spinal joint or disk. The doctor would also check your knee and ankle reflexes to see whether the nerves to the leg are functioning properly. To rule out a vascular problem, the doctor might check the pulses in your legs and feet.

If you do not have leg pain and your back pain has been present for only a few days, your doctor might wait a few weeks before ordering an x-ray exam, since most simple back strains will resolve within a month. If there are no mechanical signs of joint or muscle dysfunction, your doctor will take your temperature to determine if you might have a fever caused by infection. When sciatica or leg pain is present, an x-ray examination might be done to rule out bony spurs or tumors, an abdominal aortic aneurysm, or some other problem that might be potentially serious or require special treatment. Thinning of a disk space without associated spur formation and other degenerative changes that take years to form may indicate recent collapse or herniation of a disk.

Sciatic leg pain that persists no matter how the leg is positioned, has been present four weeks or longer, or is accompanied by loss of sensation, bladder or bowel function changes, or muscle weakness that interferes with heel-walking, toe-walking, or squatting, may indicate a need for an MRI (magnetic resonance imaging), a CT scan (computerized tomography), or a visit to a neurologist or a neurosurgeon. Electromyography and related tests may be used to locate damaged nerves and to determine the severity of the problem. The algorithms in Appendix C indicate when these various studies should be done.

Getting Treatment

If simple back pain (without sciatic or leg pain) has not subsided after two or three days of rest, physical therapy or spinal manipulation might be useful in relieving symptoms. If no danger signs are present, special testing may not be required unless symptoms last more than a month.

After two to four days of rest or refraining from exertion, you should try to resume light activities. Prolonged bed rest (more than four days) may do more harm than good and lead to weakness and debilitation.

Your physician can determine from your history if you might need blood work or special testing to rule out arthritis, infection, or tumors. An orthopedic specialist or a chiropractor might be recommended for unrelieved mechanical-type back pain.

If your doctor determines that manipulation or physical therapy is appropriate treatment for your back pain, you might be referred to a chiropractor, physical therapist, or osteopathic physician. Manipulation is often more effective than physical therapy in relieving the symptoms of simple, uncomplicated back pain. But such treatment should be discontinued after one month if no improvement results.

Acetaminophen (Tylenol) and nonsteroidal anti-inflammatory over-the-counter drugs such as aspirin are often safer and just as effective as prescription drugs in relieving uncomplicated back pain.

During the first few days after any back injury, it's always best and safer to use cold rather than heat, since cold tends to reduce swelling and inflammation. Judicious use of cold and heat is often an effective treatment option when used in self-administered home programs.

Ultrasound, which uses high-frequency sound waves to generate heat in deep tissues, is commonly used by doctors to treat back pain. When muscles are involved, electrical stimulation is often used to relax tight muscles and to relieve pain by modifying pain perception. Ultrasound and electrical stimulation are sometimes used together to ease pain and muscle spasm.

Diathermy, which uses shortwave radio waves to generate heat, is sometimes used to treat chronic back pain. Persons with diabetic neuropathy and other disorders (such as damage to a spinal nerve) that result in loss of skin sensation must be careful to avoid burns from excessive diathermy.

Massage is often helpful in relieving muscle pain and spasm. But a patient must be cautious to avoid "trigger point goading" when such treatment increases pain by bruising and irritating muscle fibers. I have seen damage occur to brachial plexus nerves by overzealous goading of the trapezius muscle near the neck.

Once you have recovered from an episode of back pain, an exercise program that includes such activities as walking, biking, or swimming would be helpful in conditioning your body and your back. Your doctor might prescribe special exercises to strengthen the supporting muscles in your lower back. Back supports, usually referred to as a lumbar support, are not often indicated but might be of some value in protecting a bad back during heavy lifting or during prolonged exertion. Shoe lifts might be helpful in relieving chronically mild back pain in individuals who have more than three-quarters of an inch difference in leg length. Older persons whose spine has compensated for leg inequality may not be able to tolerate a shoe lift. Shoe-lift use should be continued only if it makes you feel better.

There is no evidence to support the use of needle injections into trigger points and ligaments. Facet or spinal joint injections can result in rare but potentially serious complications and do not appear to be effective for treating low-back problems [27]. Acupuncture or dry needling (use of needles without mediation) has not been proven effective against low-back pain.

It is always best to use conservative methods before resorting to invasive needle procedures unless back or leg pain is so intractable that surgery is being considered. Corticosteroids, anesthetics, or narcotics are sometimes injected into epidural spaces around painful spinal nerves to relieve swelling, inflammation, and pain in an effort to avoid spinal surgery.

Choosing a Doctor

When back pain occurs for the first time, it is generally a good idea to see your family physician to rule out disease and infection that might be causing your pain. Your doctor can then refer you to an appropriate specialist if necessary. Most doctors will refer you to an orthopedist if your back pain is mechanical in origin or to a neurologist or a neurosurgeon if sciatic-type leg pain or numbness is present. If spinal manipulation is indicated, you might be referred to a chiropractor. Some physical therapists are now performing spinal manipulation.

Once it has been established that your back pain is of the mechanical, uncomplicated variety, you can seek chiropractic care on your own or by referral. But you must be prepared to deal with the nonsense that is so often associated with chiropractic treatment. When you and your physician have identified a rational chiropractor who uses spinal manipulation appropriately, it would be reasonable to see that chiropractor first for back pain that is not severe and appears to have resulted from a simple strain or injury. A competent chiropractor would know when to refer you to a medical specialist.

What Is Spinal Manipulation?

Spinal manipulation is a forceful, high-velocity thrust that stretches a joint beyond its passive range of movement in order to increase mobility (range of motion). Sudden appearance of back pain with loss of normal movement after an awkward or unprotected movement may be an indication of "joint locking" that can benefit from manipulation. A gradual onset of stiffness following recovery from a spinal injury may signal the development of adhesions as a result of formation of fibrous tissue in and around the injured joints. Prolonged immobilization of the spine following injury, fractures, or surgery can result in loss of normal lubricating (synovial) fluid between joint surfaces, decreasing the voluntary range of motion. Inactivity, postural defects, curvatures, and abnormal joint structure may cause joint dysfunction or stiffness as a result of lack of normal movement and impaired joint lubrication. These types of problems can be helped by manipulation that forces joints to move through a full range of movement and a little beyond, stretching or tearing fibrous tissue and opening joint surfaces for improved lubrication. Back pain caused by strain or sprain can often by relieved by manipulation that disperses accumulated tissue fluids around injured joints if not performed too soon after the injury.

To examine for loss of mobility, the examining doctor may have the patient bend and move in certain directions in order to detect lack of movement between spinal segments. Feeling the bony processes of the vertebrae during active movement may reveal loss of movement between two or more segments. Chiropractors call this examination procedure "motion palpation."

Of course, when an acute locked back occurs, the pain and spasm produce obvious signs of loss of movement in a joint on one side of the spine. Unlocking a locked joint with manipulation produces dramatic and immediate results, whereas manipulation to restore normal movement in a joint stiffened by adhesions may be uncomfortable, and full recovery may take many weeks.

X-ray examinations are rarely helpful in locating joints that will benefit from manipulation. Imaging procedures are useful for identifying disk herniation nerve-root encroachment for which manipulation may be inappropriate. The patient's history and the physical examination usually indicate what needs to be done.

Hands-on spinal manipulation involves use of the hands in actual pushing, stretching, and rotation of spinal structures in certain directions, depending upon the type of problem the patient has and the structure of the joint or joints being manipulated. For

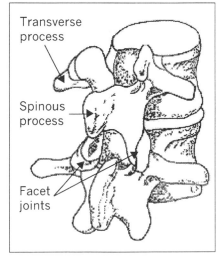

Transverse process

Spinous process

Facet joints

Rear view of two vertebrae

example, a thoracic vertebra can be manipulated or loosened by placing the heel of the hand over a transverse process on one side of the spine while anchoring the opposite side with the opposite hand. With the patient face-down on a special table and the doctor standing over the patient with both hands on the patient's back, gentle pressure is applied until downward movement ceases. Then, while the patient exhales to remove the cushion effect of air in the lungs, a sudden but shallow downward and headward thrust is made, with a little twist, to move the joint in question upward. This is an example of short-lever manipulation, which is used when the problem is confined to only one joint.

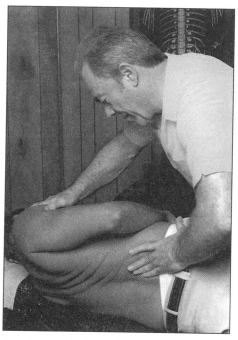

Lumbar manipulation is effective against some types of back pain but should not be repeated if it is painful or aggravates sciatic-type leg pain.

When more than one joint is involved, a "long lever" technique may be used so that several joints can be loosened simultaneously. This is typically done with both hands, with the thumb side of each hand placed over the transverse processes of two or three vertebrae. Such thrusting may be repeated up and down the spine until general loosening is accomplished. The direction of movement is different in different portions of the spine, requiring that manipulation conform to the angle of the joint surfaces. So there are a variety of manipulative techniques that can be used to stretch, rotate, or move joints in various directions.

In the area of the lumbar spine and pelvis, rotation is commonly used to move or mobilize one or more vertebrae. With the patient in a side posture position, for example, the heel of the hand may be placed over a portion of the sacrum, the pelvis, or a specific vertebra in order to apply pressure or to thrust in a corrective direction. If the object is simply to loosen all the lumbar vertebrae, hand pressure may be applied on one side of the lower back, with the opposite hand bracing the patient's shoulder, while the spine is being rotated in a side-posture position. Stretching with additional forced rotation of the lumbar spine may result in several pops when the joint surfaces separate. This is another example of long-lever manipulation.

When tight or binding joints are loosened to restore normal mobility, muscle spasm subsides and restoration of joint lubrication in a previously immobile joint reduces irritation between joint surfaces. A truly binding spinal joint can often be released with one manipulation, making further treatment unnecessary.

Properly performed scientific spinal manipulation is always done by hand. Science-based practitioners usually limit its use to treatment of mechanical-type problems in spinal joints. Pain, loss of mobility, and other symptoms in these joints can often be relieved by loosening the involved joints and stretching tight muscles. Some chiropractors who "adjust" the spine to restore and maintain health by correcting "vertebral subluxations" may use a handheld, spring-loaded mallet to tap a selected vertebra "back into alignment." Such instrument adjusting is not an acceptable substitute for hands-on manipulation in the treatment of back pain (see Chapter 10).

Several research teams have evaluated the published studies testing the effectiveness of spinal manipulation against low-back pain. In 1991, based on an analysis of twenty-two controlled studies, a RAND Corporation panel concluded that manipulation was useful for acute low-back pain in patients showing no signs of lower-limb nerve-root involvement [165]. An appropriate trial, the report said, would be two weeks each of two different types of manipulation, after which, if there is no improvement, therapy should be discontinued. In 1994, the Agency for Health Care Policy and Research (AHCPR) concluded that, "For patients with acute low-back pain symptoms without radiculopathy [nerve injury], the scientific evidence suggests spinal manipulation is effective in reducing pain and perhaps speeding recovery within the first month of symptoms" [27]. In 1996, a prominent Dutch research team evaluated thirty-six randomized clinical trials and concluded that manipulation might be effective in some subgroups of patients with low-back pain, but that the studies were not well designed and more were needed [109].

The Popping Sound

Manipulation is usually accompanied by an audible pop or click. This may occur when a locked joint is unlocked, but it can also occur with a normal joint. The joint surfaces (facets) that connect two vertebrae fit together like two wet glass slides. The facets slide freely upon each other to allow movement of the vertebrae, but they normally do not separate. The surface tension of the fluid between the joint surfaces holds the facets together. When manipulation forcefully separates them, the resultant vacuum pulls in nitrogen gas to fill the space, producing a pop, much like the popping of a cork. The technical term for this is "cavitation." Once the joint pops, it may be a few hours before the gas is absorbed and the joint surfaces settle back together so that cavitation can recur during manipulation. The popping sound can have considerable placebo effect.

The fact that a joint pops does not mean that anything was out of place. Unfortunately, many people who get regular chiropractic adjustments believe that it does, and some unethical chiropractors encourage this belief so their patients will keep coming for "maintenance" care. Patients who believe that their vertebrae keep slipping in and out of place can become psychologically addicted to spinal manipulation and may be dissatisfied if they do not hear a pop during manipulation. Dr. James Cyriax, a prominent English orthopedic surgeon who specialized in the use of manipulation, called this dependency "chiropractogenic neurosis" and discussed it in his *Textbook of Orthopedic Medicine* [53].

Chiropractors who believe that a pop signals replacement of a subluxated vertebra may tend to use as much force as necessary to elicit the coveted pop. This obsession with popping the vertebrae has resulted in more than one broken rib, especially in elderly persons who have calcium-deficient bones.

Reasons Not to Have Spinal Manipulation

The AHCPR guidelines list these "red flags" as contraindications to using spinal manipulation to treat acute back pain:

- Cancer or infection, which might be suggested by history of cancer, unexplained weight loss, immunosuppression, urinary infection, fever, intravenous drug use, prolonged use of corticosteroids, back pain not improved with rest, and age of patient over fifty.

- Spinal or compression fracture, which might be suggested by history of significant trauma in the case of a young adult, or back pain following a minor fall or exertion in the case of an elderly person who might have osteoporosis, prolonged use of steroids, and age over seventy.

- Cauda equina syndrome, as might be suggested by sudden onset of urinary retention or overflow (incontinence), loss of anal sphincter tone or fecal incontinence, saddle anesthesia (numbness or loss of sensation in the area of the anus, perineum, and genitals), and global or progressive weakness in the lower limbs.

- Herniated disk, as suggested by sciatica (pain radiating down one leg below the knee), which might be increased when the affected leg is raised up in front while the knee is locked out straight. Manipulation of a herniated lumbar disk could produce cauda equina syndrome.

- Spinal stenosis (narrowing of the spinal canal), as suggested by weakness and cramping in both legs, unaffected by straight leg raising, and age over fifty.

- Ankylosing spondylitis, as suggested by low-back pain not relieved by rest, stiffness in the morning with persistent pain lasting longer than three months in persons under the age of forty.

If you have back or leg pain and red flags are present, always see your family physician before considering chiropractic treatment. A simple lab test such as a urinalysis, blood cell count, or a red cell sedimentation rate might provide clues of a need for referral to a medical specialist for more extensive testing.

Additional Cautions

Persons over the age of seventy should be cautious about submitting to spinal manipulation lest they have undetected osteoporosis (weak, porous bones). A bone density examination may reveal osteoporosis that is not evident on plain x-rays. (Osteoporosis does not show on plain x-ray films until a 40 percent bone loss has occurred.)

Osteoporotic collapse of a lumbar vertebra is not always evident in postural exams. Collapse or fracture of a vertebra in the thoracic spine can result in the sudden appearance of a painful hump in the upper back. While this happens most often in women, it is not rare in men. Manipulation should never be used in such cases or when x-ray examination reveals the presence of a crush fracture.

When back pain is severe and is accompanied by pain that radiates into the calf or foot, with numbness or tingling, there may be nerve-root compression caused by disk herniation. Your family physician might want to order a CT scan or an MRI exam. It's not a good idea to delay seeing a doctor when leg pain is present, even if only for a few days. According to federal guidelines, spinal manipulation is contraindicated when there is sciatica or leg pain [27]. Anecdotal evidence indicates that spinal manipulation will sometimes relieve leg pain that is associated with back pain, but if symptoms are made worse by manipulation, the treatment should not be repeated.

In the case of back pain, spinal manipulations should not be continued for longer than one month if no improvement results. A competent chiropractor will not hesitate to refer you to an orthopedist or a neurologist for a second opinion if symptoms persist longer than two weeks or if the pain worsens after a few days.

Some chiropractors pad their income by recommending unnecessary procedures. Daily spinal manipulation is rarely necessary, and twice-a-day manipulation is never a good idea. Padding can also occur with heat treatments. Ultrasound, diathermy, hot packs, and whirlpool baths may play a useful role in managing back pain. Their action is similar enough, however, that one modality is usually sufficient and more than two are never necessary during the same visit.

Since chiropractors are not licensed to prescribe medication, you will have to rely upon a physician to prescribe pain pills if needed. Fortunately, over-the-counter medications such as acetaminophen, aspirin, and other nonsteroidal anti-inflammatory drugs may be just as effective as prescription medication in relieving simple back pain [27].

Spinal manipulation should not be painful and should not be used if it causes pain. Some chiropractors tell their patients that a painful reaction to spinal manipulation is a sign that the body is "retracing" symptoms, that is, the condition must get worse before it gets better. This is nonsense. If a manipulation is painful, or if it makes your symptoms worse, it is either inappropriate or improperly performed. Loss of bowel or bladder control following a lumbar manipulation would require emergency care by a neurosurgeon. Fortunately, it is rare.

Don't submit to repeated manipulation that makes you hurt worse. I have seen patients who went to a chiropractor for "preventive maintenance" spinal adjustments and experienced back pain after each session. They continued to return for more, however, because they felt that pain was a natural result of getting misaligned vertebrae back in place. Additional treatment may then be given for the symptoms caused by the manipulation.

Scoliosis Management

Scoliosis, in which two side-to-side spinal curves form an "S" shape, is not often a cause of back pain. Adults who have curvatures that measure less than 20 degrees do not usually have symptoms and rarely need treatment of any kind. Most people have some spinal curvature, often as a result of leg-length inequality, which is common, or a structural abnormality of spinal or pelvic joints. Most persons who have abnormal spinal curves are not aware of them. Curvatures that measure 10 degrees or less are considered to be within normal limits. Curvatures that measure more than 20 degrees might eventually cause spinal arthritis and other joint and muscle symptoms as a result of imbalances in posture and weightbearing. Adults who have backache caused by such curvatures can often obtain symptomatic relief from manipulation, exercise, and physical therapy. But these do not straighten out the curvatures.

If you have a spinal curvature that causes no symptoms, you do not need treatment of any kind—other than some regular exercise to maintain the tone of your back muscles. If you do have back pain caused by a scoliosis or a hump in your back, your chiropractor may be able to provide symptomatic relief. But don't continue treatment when you are symptom-free. And don't go to chiropractors who say that they can correct a structural scoliosis in anyone over the age of sixteen. Once full growth has been reached, curvatures have usually reached their maximum level of deformity, except for severe cases where childhood idiopathic scoliosis has progressed to 50 or 60 degrees.

Unfortunately, some chiropractors take advantage of the fact that many adults have abnormal curves in their spine. Chiropractors who conduct posture-screening exams in malls, schools, and other public places often label harmless and insignificant curvature as a potential problem that can have damaging effects by producing subluxations in the spine. The evaluation may include measurements made on a twin-scale device called a spinal analysis machine (see Chapter 8). Many people with harmless spinal curvatures are frightened into undergoing long courses of chiropractic adjustments to "correct or prevent progression" of the curvatures—even if they have no symptoms.

Scoliosis in children, especially the idiopathic variety that grows progressively worse without bracing or surgery, should always be brought to the attention of an orthopedic specialist. A scoliosis caused by unequal leg length or by a skeletal abnormality may show up between six and ten years of age and will develop into a permanent structural scoliosis if not corrected early. An idiopathic scoliosis, which develops for no apparent reason, may become evident between ten and twelve years of age. When a curvature begins to progress beyond 20 degrees in a child who is still growing, a brace or surgery may be advisable. Curvatures that are allowed to progress to as much as 50 or 60 degrees may continue to progress, even after the child stops growing, causing crippling deformity and life-threatening compression of vital organs.

Spinal manipulation cannot prevent or correct idiopathic scoliosis. This condition should be kept under observation by an orthopedic specialist, who might refer the child to a surgeon who specializes in the treatment of juvenile scoliosis. Parents who rely on chiropractic care when medical care is needed may wind up with a child who is permanently deformed.

Inappropriate Manipulation: An Instructive Case

Although spinal manipulation is often beneficial in the treatment of back pain, some chiropractors aggravate back pain with excessive and inappropriate use of spinal adjustments to correct "subluxations" or to "realign the vertebrae." I have seen patients who had such excessive manipulation in a chiropractor's office that they were nearly incapacitated with acute back pain.

I remember one patient in particular, Clyde, who visited my office without an appointment. He was on crutches and was on his way to see an orthopedist for "back surgery." His pain was limited to his lower back, and had no sciatic nerve symptoms that would indicate a possible disk protrusion.

When questioned, Clyde told me that he initially had minor back pain that had gotten worse after several visits to his chiropractor. He explained that the chiropractor adjusted his spine daily and then increased the frequency to *twice* daily when his pain worsened. The chiropractor told Clyde that the frequent treatment was necessary to keep his vertebrae in proper alignment, because the adjustments were not "holding" (keeping the "subluxated" vertebrae in place). The treatments continued until Clyde was unable to walk without crutches. The chiropractor then told Clyde that he needed back surgery and made him an appointment with an out-of-town orthopedic surgeon. It was on the day of that scheduled appointment that Clyde dropped by my office.

After obtaining Clyde's history, examining his back, and performing a neurological examination, I told him that it was possible that his back had been aggravated by excessive manipulation and that the best treatment might be to discontinue manipulation and rest at home. About a week later, he walked into my office without crutches and with minimal pain. His symptoms, which were apparently the result of excessive and inappropriate manipulation, simply subsided with time—and no additional treatment.

Some chiropractors have a tendency to overmanipulate back pain under the false assumption that every patient has a vertebra out of place. Often, what they interpret as a subluxated vertebra is simply structural asymmetry that is insignificant and can't be altered by spinal manipulation. Attempts to "realign" such vertebrae in patients who have acute back pain can only cause trouble. In this respect, a chiropractor's belief in subluxations as an underlying cause of disease can overshadow the benefits of appropriate manipulation.

Some Final Advice

Because spinal manipulation is not readily available in medical practice, many people visit chiropractors seeking manipulation for back pain. The problem is finding a rational, properly limited chiropractor who will use spinal manipulation appropriately. Consumers who are well informed about questionable practices in chiropractic have a better chance of finding a rational chiropractor and getting appropriate treatment.

If spinal manipulation feels good and you enjoy the treatment, it's okay to get such treatment when you experience obvious benefits. But you should not go for regular spinal manipulation if you are under the impression that "keeping your spine in line" will keep you healthy and prevent disease. In other words, stop the treatment when the pain is gone. Return for treatment only if the pain recurs. Remember the old adage, "If it ain't broke, don't fix it."

7

Neck and Head
Problems

Neck pain is as common as back pain but can be more difficult to treat. The cervical spine permits movement of the head in all directions. Because its structures are complicated and delicate, neck manipulation is potentially more dangerous and must be performed more carefully and specifically than manipulation of other areas of the spine. Muscle-tension headaches and shoulder, arm, and hand pain are commonly associated with mechanical-type neck problems, such as herniation of a cervical disk, osteophyte (spur) formation, and muscle tension caused by postural strain or other factors. A competent chiropractor can do much to help with these problems, but inappropriate treatment can do more harm than good.

The RAND report on *The Appropriateness of Manipulation and Mobilization of the Cervical Spine,* released in 1996, concluded that cervical manipulation or mobilization may improve range of motion and provide short-term relief for subacute or chronic neck pain and muscle-tension headache [49]. One part of the study involved listing and rating the reasons why chiropractors do neck manipulation. Of 736 reported "indications," RAND's expert panel rated 424 (57.6 percent) as inappropriate, 230 (31.3 percent) as uncertain, and 82 (11.1 percent) as appropriate. Since no data were available on the relative frequency of use of these procedures, the panel drew no conclusions about the percentage of manipulations that fit these categories. However, it is safe to assume that a large percentage of chiropractic neck manipulations are not medically justifiable.

Neck massage, which provides a safer alternative, can be as effective as cervical spine manipulation in relieving episodic or recurring tension-type headaches [30]. Most chiropractors can perform neck massage, but it can also be done at home with a little instruction. Some forms of chronic headache caused by loss of mobility in the joints of the cervical spine (producing a cervicogenic headache) can be permanently relieved with appropriate manipulation. If massage does not relieve a chronic headache, neck manipulation or mobilization might make sense provided that a medical examination has ruled out any serious or potential problems.

Although the RAND report supported the use of manipulation for treating neck pain and muscle-tension headache, it concluded that there is not sufficient evidence to support or refute using it and/or mobilization for migraine headache or shoulder-arm-hand pain referred from the neck. Like low-back pain with associated sciatica or nerve-root involvement, head or shoulder-arm-hand pain resulting from encroachment upon cervical spinal nerves may not be an appropriate indication for cervical manipulation. You should be cautious when considering use of cervical manipulation for an actual pinched nerve in your neck. When shoulder, arm, or hand pain is made worse by cervical manipulation, the treatment should not be repeated.

How the Neck Is Constructed

There are seven cervical vertebrae. As in other portions of the spine, these vertebrae are aligned by interlocking facets, separated and cushioned by tough cartilage (intervertebral disks), and held together by strong ligaments. However, the cervical spine has one unique feature: its top two vertebrae do not have intervertebral disks and their shapes permit greater rotation, which is needed to turn the head. This makes the cervical spine more susceptible to serious injury. The region of the atlas (the topmost vertebra that supports the skull) and axis (the vertebra that supports the atlas) is most vulnerable to accidental injury and inappropriate cervical manipulation. Their

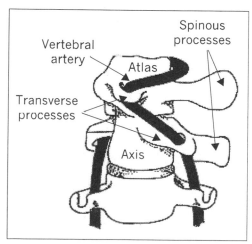

Front view showing how extreme rotation of the atlas stretches the left vertebral artery where it passes through a transverse process.

dislocation in a severe injury, for example, can compress or sever the brain stem, causing total body paralysis and respiratory failure. Inappropriate cervical manipulation that forces excessive rotation of the head and atlas can cause a stroke by damaging the vertebral arteries that pass through bony channels on each side of the vertebrae to carry blood to the brain. Overly vigorous manipulation can also injure one of the carotid arteries that pass through the soft tissues of the neck to supply blood to structures of the head, face, and neck.

Causes of Neck and Arm Pain

Most neck problems, like low-back problems, result from strain, sprain, degenerative changes, or disk herniation. And as with low-back problems, encroachment upon spinal nerves in the neck is most often the result of disk herniation or degenerative changes that cause spur formation or narrowing of openings between the vertebrae. Slight misalignment of a cervical vertebra is rarely significant.

After age fifty, cervical disk degeneration with associated bony spur formation (often called spondylosis) is a common cause of neck pain or loss of mobility. Simple muscle tension is a common cause of neck pain. Many of my former patients had neck pain from muscle inflammation caused by prolonged tension on neck muscles as a result of job stress. Bookkeepers, dentists, hairdressers, and computer operators, for example, are often victims of job-related soreness and stiffness in neck muscles.

Acute spasm of neck muscles is less common, but when it does occur as a "crick" in the neck, it will often resolve after four or five days without treatment. When neck spasm lasts longer than a week, the cervical spine should be examined carefully. In some cases, a joint in the cervical spine will lock and can be released with a single cervical manipulation, resulting in immediate relief of symptoms.

Persistent neck pain caused by disk herniation, however, especially when accompanied by nerve pain in the arm, might be aggravated by cervical manipulation. Severe neck injuries, such as those that can occur in an auto accident (whiplash), on a football field, or in a headfirst fall should be checked by an orthopedic specialist, reserving any use of manipulation for a later date. Immobilization of the cervical spine or use of a cervical collar is sometimes necessary during the first few weeks following a severe neck injury.

Signs and Symptoms

A doctor can often tell whether neck pain has a musculoskeletal cause by comparing the effects of active and passive movement of the head and neck. When bone disease or disk herniation is suspected, an x-ray examination might be indicated, which might then point to the need for an MRI, a CT scan, a bone scan, or some other high-tech diagnostic procedure. Unrelieved symptoms that could be caused by infection or a malignancy may require other laboratory testing. It is important to rule out disk herniation or serious disease before accepting a diagnosis of "arthritis" or "myofascitis" when you are told that you must live with your neck pain.

When a cervical nerve is pinched, it is usually not difficult to determine which spinal segment is involved. The location of pain, weakness, numbness, and other symptoms in the head, neck, shoulder, arm, and hand will correspond to the nerves that emerge between the segments:

C1	Top of head
C2, C3	Back of the head and around the neck
C4	Across the shoulders and upper back
C5	Upper arm
C6	Thumb, first finger, and forearm
C7	Long finger
C8	Ring finger and the little finger

If necessary, a neurologist can test muscle function and nerve conduction speed with tests in which small needle electrodes are used to detect electrical activity.

Weakness or shrinkage in muscles supplied by pinched or irritated spinal nerves, or loss of deep tendon reflexes in the area of the pain and numbness, are signs of nerve damage, most often the result of disk herniation or spur formation. A damaged C4 nerve, for example, can weaken a shoulder muscle, making it difficult to lift the arm on that side. Such weakness should not be confused with inability to lift because of painful bursitis or tendinitis, which causes pain on movement. Damage to nerves supplying the shoulder muscles will result in weakness but no pain on movement. A compressed nerve in the lower part of the cervical spine (C6 to C8), which can weaken the handgrip, must be differentiated from carpal tunnel syndrome, which originates in the wrist. This can usually be determined by checking reflexes at the elbow and examining the wrist and hand for evidence of carpal tunnel nerve compression. In some cases, an enlarged neck muscle or an extra rib on the lowest cervical vertebra can compress blood vessels and nerves in the neck, causing symptoms that affect the entire arm—a condition called thoracic outlet syndrome. A scientifically oriented chiropractor can help deal with these problems, but if nerve damage progresses to the point where there is muscle weakness or loss of reflexes, a neurologist or neurosurgeon should be consulted.

Many chiropractors place unwarranted importance upon slight deviations from normal in the cervical spine, basing prolonged treatment upon insignificant findings. The normal cervical spine curves toward the front of the neck. Occasionally, however, this curve flattens or is reversed. This abnormality can result from degeneration or herniation of cervical intervertebral disks or from postural influences. Most often, however, it is a normal compensation for joint irregularity or a spinal curvature, such as scoliosis. Compensatory curves do not usually cause trouble and cannot be corrected. They should not be manipulated if they are not causing symptoms. Yet, some chiropractors will prescribe long courses of treatment to "restore the normal cervical curve," which may be futile, unnecessary, and even harmful.

Neck Manipulation Cautions

All chiropractors perform neck manipulation, some more than others. Although scientific studies support limited usage, techniques that combine too much rotation with extension of the cervical spine should not be used, and some people should not have their neck manipulated at all. Properly performed cervical manipulation can loosen or mobilize vertebrae with a minimum amount of rotation and without tilting the head backward, which extends the cervical spine. Some techniques entail little or no rotation or extension, including those that employ manipulative traction. But when cervical rotation is needed to restore range of motion in vertebrae stiffened by adhesions, fixations, or binding of cervical facet joints, it should be done with less than 50 degrees of head rotation. This can be accomplished by placing one hand on each side of the neck (rather than the head) while the patient sits on a stool. With the head tilted slightly forward and slightly flexed, the neck is rotated and given a quick tug at the end of the rotation. This enables neck joints to be loosened with less than the patient's normal active cervical rotation.

Injury from neck manipulation is usually the result of extreme rotation in which the practitioner's hands are placed on the patient's head in order to rotate the cervical spine by rotating the head. This occurs most often when the patient is lying on his back to permit forced, passive rotation of the head, which twists and strains the vertebral arteries.

Two recent reports have examined the issue of neck manipulation and safety. In 1996, the National Chiropractic Mutual Insurance Company, which is the largest American chiropractic malpractice insurer, published a report called *Vertebrobasilar Stroke Following Manipulation*, written by Allen G.J. Terrett, an Australian chiropractic educator/researcher. Terrett based his findings on 183 cases of vertebrobasilar strokes (VBS) reported between 1934 and 1994. He concluded that 105 of the manipulations had been administered by a chiropractor, twenty-five were done by a medical practitioner, thirty-one had been done by another type of practitioner, and that the practitioner type for the remaining twenty-two was not specified in the report. He concluded that VBS is "very rare," that current pretesting procedures are seldom able to predict susceptibility, and that in twenty-five cases serious injury might have been avoided if the practitioner had recognized that symptoms occurring after a manipulation indicated that further manipulations should not be done. Here are two examples from Dr. Terrett's report:

> Case 2. Following manipulation the patient said "Oh, that was awful, something terrible has happened to me. That's awful. Let me up. I don't want any more; I can't stand any more." The chiropractor then said "you will be all right. Let me get this other one." The patient then said "I have had enough, don't, stop." The chiropractor continued to manipulate the patient. Immediately following the adjustment she was unable to walk, her vision was impaired, she vomited, and she had a partial paralysis of the throat and vocal cords.

> Case 3. The chiropractor manipulated the neck both to the right and to the left. The patient screamed, then said several times "I'm falling," but the chiropractor continued to manipulate her neck. The patient was then helped to a chair by her husband and the chiropractor. She could not hold her head up, her face and hands were numb, she began to vomit and suffered convulsions. The patient died 18 hours later. [186]

The 1996 RAND report, *The Appropriateness of Manipulation and Mobilization of the Cervical Spine,* tabulated more than a hundred published case reports and estimated that the number of strokes, cord compressions, fractures, and large blood clots was 1.46 per million neck manipulations. Even though this number appears small, it is significant because many of the manipulations chiropractors do should not be done. In addition, as the report itself noted, neither the number of manipulations performed nor the number of complications has been systematically studied [49]. Since some people are more susceptible than others, it has also been argued that the incidence should be expressed as rate per patient rather than rate per adjustment.

Chiropractors cannot agree among themselves whether the VBS problem is significant enough to inform patients that neck manipulation is a possible complication of manipulation. I believe it is and that the profession should devise a reporting system that would enable this matter to be appropriately studied. This might be achieved if (a) state licensing boards required that all such cases be reported, and (b) chiropractic malpractice insurance companies, which now keep their data secret, were required to disclose them.

Most people with neck pain who go to a chiropractor will be advised to undergo manipulation. Unless you consult a scientifically directed chiropractor, you may have to be alert to avoid inappropriate treatment. Persons with active cervical rheumatoid arthritis, for example, should avoid cervical manipulation. Rheumatoid arthritis can destroy joints and cartilage to such an extent that the atlas can slip forward on the axis. Manipulation of such a neck could be very dangerous. People over the age of seventy

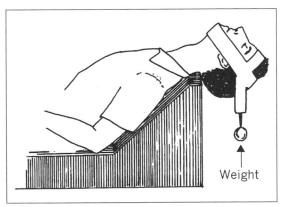

Weight

Some chiropractors use a traction-extension treatment purported to increase the curvature of the cervical spine. Sustained, forced hyperextension of the cervical spine is an abnormal posture that can interfere with blood flow in carotid and vertebral arteries and encroach upon spinal nerves. Cervical traction is normally performed with a slight amount of neck flexion or stretching. Forced hyperextension to "restore the normal cervical curve" may be futile as well as dangerous.

should probably avoid neck manipulation, because their vertebral arteries may be more brittle and prone to damage. Anticoagulant therapy is another contraindication.

Before neck manipulation is performed, the carotid arteries should be examined for evidence of partial blockage. This is done by placing a stethoscope over the neck to listen for murmurs that may indicate that blood flow through the carotid arteries is restricted. Vascular insufficiency in the more protected vertebral arteries can sometimes be detected by observing the effects of combining head rotation with extension of the neck. In any event, treatment of the cervical spine, whether by manipulation, traction, or massage, requires careful attention to the status of blood vessels as well as bone structure. And note should be made of any disease process or medication (such as anticoagulants) that might contribute to increased bleeding in a damaged artery.

Manipulation of the cervical spine should be done only when specifically indicated—after a careful diagnosis has been made and contraindications have been ruled out. Techniques in which head rotation is used as leverage to rotate the cervical spine should be avoided. No matter who proposes to manipulate your neck, ask for an explanation and make sure that extreme cervical rotation is not used. You do not have to submit to any treatment without your consent. You certainly should not submit to a second neck manipulation following an adverse reaction of any type. Most strokes caused by cervical manipulation occur when a second manipulation is performed after the patient has complained of ill effects.

Some chiropractors believe that most human ailments are the result of misalignment of the atlas and axis and that every patient they see needs neck manipulation. Unnecessary manipulation of the atlas, in the area where manipulation is most dangerous, is not uncommon in chiropractic offices. You should refuse treatment by any type of chiropractic "upper cervical specialist." (See Chapter 11.)

Other Approaches

Some chiropractors combine cervical manipulation with physical therapy for neck pain. A physical therapist might combine cervical mobilization with physical therapy. Osteopaths, physiatrists, and other practitioners might combine manipulation with massage, neck traction, ultrasound, electrical stimulation, and other forms of physical therapy.

In many cases, home care can be beneficial. Stubborn cases of neck pain can sometimes benefit from use of cervical traction at home. Moist heat or cold packs might be helpful. Most of the time, however, moist heat, such as a hot shower over the back of the neck, or a hot, wet compress, is very effective. A good rule of thumb is to use cold for three or four days following a severe injury or sprain, since cold constricts blood vessels and reduces bleeding and swelling. Early use of heat might increase swelling by increasing blood flow. Once pain and swelling have subsided, moist heat can speed healing by increasing circulation. Furthermore, use of moist heat on chronic neck problems helps increase the range of motion by warming and increasing pliability of neck structures. Chronic neck arthritis, for example, usually always responds better to moist heat than to cold packs. Before beginning any form of home treatment, you should seek the advice of a doctor who can tell you what your problem is and what you should do.

Although spinal traction is no longer used much for low-back pain, many doctors still recommend neck traction for certain types of neck pain, especially when there is shoulder or arm and hand pain caused by nerve-root encroachment in the cervical spine. Use of such treatment should always be prescribed by a doctor and should not be used if it increases pain.

Injured or inflamed joints and ligaments can be aggravated by sustained neck stretching. In some cases, neck traction can increase encroachment upon a swollen spinal nerve. If manual cervical traction relieves neck or arm pain, then there is a good possibility you could benefit from use of cervical traction at home. Many drugstores and orthopedic supply companies can supply a cervical traction apparatus that can be used while lying in bed or sitting up.

People tend to rely upon the judgment of the first practitioner they consult and may not be inclined to question the treatment. However, if neck pain does not improve after two or three treatments or worsens even after one treatment, you should seek a second opinion from a medical specialist.

Finally, although vertebral artery injury is not common, you should know how to recognize the symptoms of this complication. If, after a neck manipulation, you experience nausea, blurred vision, dizziness, difficulty in swallowing, mental dullness, or head pain, seek immediate medical care (preferably at a hospital emergency room) and inform the doctor that the problem followed a neck manipulation.

8

Questionable
Marketing Strategies

Susan B, a department store clerk, was forty-one years old when she first visited my office, complaining of back pain, which was caused by muscle spasm triggered by inflammation of an arthritic joint in her lumbar spine. During the next four years, she saw me several times. All she needed was gentle manipulation or mobilization along with ultrasound, electrical stimulation, or some other type of physical therapy. After a few treatments, she would be fine for several months—until she reinjured her back. She would then call for another appointment.

A few months after Susan's last visit, she moved to another state. When she hurt her back moving furniture, she went to a local chiropractor. That night, she called my home, obviously distressed and frightened:

> Dr. Homola, I went to a chiropractor today to get treatment for my lower back. He took x-rays of my neck and back and told me it would take three months to get them into proper alignment. He said that the top vertebra in my neck is too close to my spinal cord and that if I did not complete the full course of treatments, my spine would degenerate and my health would deteriorate. Is that possible? He wants me to pay for the treatments in advance, and he said that once he got my alignment corrected he could keep my vertebrae in place with one treatment a month. What should I do?

As I listened to this account, several things were obvious. Susan had fallen into the hands of a subluxation-based chiropractor who maintained that every spine should be checked and "adjusted" monthly. This particular chiropractor also believed that alignment of the topmost vertebra (atlas) was paramount, even for problems in the low-back area. There was no logical reason to x-ray her neck and, in fact, no good reason to x-ray her back. Nor was there any valid reason to believe that failing to achieve and maintain "spinal alignment" would have disastrous consequences. Needless to say, I advised Susan to seek care elsewhere.

Unfortunately, what happened to Susan is not rare. In fact, it is a natural consequence of subluxation theory. Spinal manipulative treatment should be provided as needed. When pain goes away, no further treatment is needed. But many chiropractors assert that periodic checkups and adjustments should be done frequently to maintain health. This chapter describes many of the strategies used to recruit patients and keep them coming back.

"Maintenance Care"

"Maintenance care"—also referred to as "preventative maintenance"—is based on the idea that early detection and correction of subluxations can promote general health and prevent many problems. Many practice-building consultants teach that the best way to build a large practice is to retain patients on a "maintenance" schedule. Patients who are in pain are not generally considered "good patients." because they usually stop coming

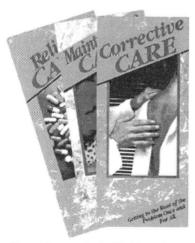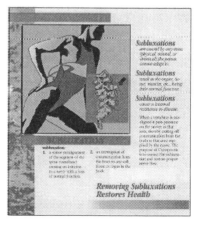

Singer Enterprise's "Subluxation" pamphlet advises that "subluxations are caused by any stress (physical, mental, or chemical) the person cannot adapt to" and "cause a lowered resistance to disease." Singer's "Corrective Care" pamphlet promises "Getting to the root of the problem once and for all" [170].

when they are pain-free. Besides, much more time is required to treat patients in pain than to service those who come for quick "preventive-maintenance" adjustments.

Singer Enterprises, a practice-building firm in Clearwater, Florida, advocates this approach in pamphlets describing three levels of care:

> Relief care is that care necessary to get rid of your symptoms or pain but not the cause of it. It is the same as drying a floor that was getting wet from a leak, but not fixing the leak. [170a]

> Corrective care is necessary not only to relieve or reduce a person's pain or symptoms, but also to remove the actual cause of the problem. . . .
> Corrective care focuses on making certain the vertebra, the cause, is corrected. . . .
> If correction is possible, it normally takes one to six months of intensive care followed by three to fifteen months of stabilization. [170b]

> Maintenance care is made necessary by the stresses of living. . . . It works to remove the cause of problems before symptoms arise or serious conditions show themselves. . . . You feel better, increase endurance and reduce the risk of health problems. [170c]

These concepts are used by mixer chiropractors as well as by straights. For example, the new-patient-orientation slide show marketed by the American Chiropractic Association labels the phases "acute care," "rehabilitative care," and "well care" [107].

The symptoms of simple back pain caused by strain will usually resolve after a few weeks. But if the patient is placed on a preventive-maintenance schedule, the treatment will last a lifetime. In many cases, it is difficult to determine whether a chiropractor really believes such long-course treatment is necessary or whether it is simply a practice-building gimmick. Regardless, there is no scientific evidence that people who feel well should undergo periodic spinal checkups or adjustments.

To my knowledge, no study has ever shown that people who have their spine checked and adjusted enjoy better health or have less disease than people who do not. In 1996, two Canadian chiropractors who had conducted an extensive search reported that "existing literature is sparse and at best anecdotal." They also concluded: (1) the belief that spinal manipulation can enhance healing is not based on scientific evidence, (2) "preventive/maintenance care" has not been precisely defined, (3) appropriate ways to measure health status have not been determined, and (4) steps 2 and 3 would be essential before valid controlled studies could be performed [2].

I think these conclusions are far too mild. Chapter 4 points out that chiropractors cannot agree on what subluxations are or how they should be diagnosed. Considering this fact, maintenance care is nonsense piled on top of nonsense.

Patient Recruitment

Chiropractors market their services in many different ways. Some rely primarily on word-of-mouth referrals from their satisfied patients and from physicians and other health professionals who respect what they do. Some engage in relatively standard public relations activities that give them public exposure. The American Chiropractic Association's practice development manual suggests such activities as holding an open house, making as many personal contacts as possible, sending out personalized mailings, participating in community affairs, offering leadership to scouting organizations and other youth groups, and presenting programs to PTA groups, civic organizations, service clubs, senior citizen groups, labor unions, and health education classes [160]. Chiropractic practice-building consultants suggest more aggressive activities such as health fair screenings, posture evaluations, patient appreciation days, telemarketing, offering free consultations, and turning one's patients into recruiters. From what I have seen, these strategies usually involve deception.

Many chiropractic offices advertise pain relief. Such newspaper or telephone book blurbs as "the pain ends here" or "get pain relief now" attract suffering patients who are then indoctrinated into a preventive-maintenance mode. It's important to understand, however, that since chiropractors do not prescribe pain medication they cannot do much to relieve severe pain. Over-the-counter medication such as aspirin or Tylenol, or use of cold packs, electrical stimulation, and other physical therapy measures, will often relieve moderate pain. But persons who are in agony should see their family physicians before seeing a chiropractor if they feel they need medication for pain relief. Some chiropractors will let their patients suffer through a "natural course of recovery" without suggesting that they consult a physician for pain medication.

Posture Screenings

Many chiropractors attract patients through free posture screenings at shopping centers, schools, health expositions, health-food stores, and their offices. Some simply look at the individual's posture and feel along the spine. Some place adhesive dots along the spine and take a Polaroid picture to show the patient whether they line up. Other chiropractors use a twin-scale device or electronic gadget. From what I have seen, virtually all who get screened are either told they have a problem (such as an abnormal curvature) or are advised to make an appointment for further evaluation.

The most commonly used "posture screening" device is the S.A.M.® Spinal Analysis Machine, which has twin scales at the base and a five-foot-high frame that has horizontal and vertical grid lines. The person being tested stands with one foot on each scale while the chiropractor records the weight readings and compares the individual's posture with the grid lines. These findings supposedly enable the chiropractor to draw conclusions about leg lengths, posture, probable areas of scoliosis, and alignment of the hips, shoulders, spine, and head. The data can be fed into a computer that issues a printed report.

The company marketing the device also provides computer software, display booths, and posters purporting to show relationships between leg-length differences, spinal curvature, "subluxations," and poor health. The posters express subluxation theory with such messages as "spinal sub-luxations can cause a lifetime of poor health," "have your family checked now. Early detection is the key to prevention."

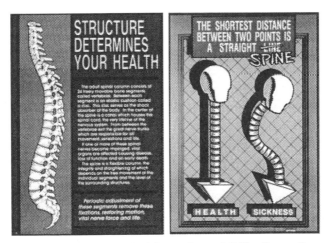

These were among a dozen "Spinal Screening and Office Posters" marketed by the S.A.M. Company in 1993. The left one claims that if one or more spinal nerves become impinged, vital organs are affected, causing disease, loss of function and an early death" and that periodic adjustment of fixated segments restores "motion, vital nerve force, and life." The company's catalog states: "Teach them about subluxation and all else becomes natural."

The computer software can generate reports describing the alleged postural imbalances, degree of "scoliosis (spinal curvature)," and a statement that most spines with scoliosis show "subluxation degeneration," which, if untreated, can progress and become irreversible. The spinal curvature is described as "probably the result of leg length deficiency" that the chiropractor can correct.

Use of the device is based on a theory that "apparent differences" in leg lengths can cause spinal curvature and subluxations, even though the leg bones are the same length. The "differences" probably reflect how the person is standing as well as normal spinal muscle tension and/or slight variations of hip position. Nevertheless the company's catalog claims that 85% of people have "apparent differences" and that use of the device can attract 20 to 40 new patients per week. One customer reported that "a recent mailing to patients produced 200 appointments for their friends to be checked on S.A.M.—nearly 100% are now under care." Another reported obtaining "96 new patients (not appointments) in one weekend."

When a nearby health fair included chiropractic "posture screening," I would receive calls from people who were told that an abnormal curvature or an "out-of-place vertebra" threatened their health. Invariably, when I examined these people, their alleged problems were either nonexistent or insignificant. I remember one woman in her mid-twenties who had been extremely frightened by a chiropractor who said that she had scoliosis that would eventually cripple her without chiropractic treatment to stop its progression. My examination found that her curvature was very slight, would not get worse, and needed no treatment. She felt instantly relieved and was very grateful for the news. "I have a new lease on life," she said.

Solicitation of Athletes

Some chiropractors are "certified" in sports medicine or in chiropractic orthopedics. While some do a good job handling sports injuries, their treatment methods differ little from those of the average chiropractor and are little more extensive than the skills of an athletic trainer. "Mixer" chiropractors who use physical therapy along with spinal manipulation are better able to handle sports injuries than "straight" chiropractors who use only spinal adjustments. However, chiropractors are not trained to reduce dislocations, set broken bones, prescribe pain medication, give injections, drain swollen knees, or perform many of the procedures that are a part of every orthopedic sports medicine practice.

Some chiropractors seek certification in sports medicine as a practice-building gimmick, drawing attention to themselves as a "team physician" for a local high school or a college athletic team. In most cases, they continue to promote the use of spinal adjustments as a method of restoring and maintaining health. Athletes treated by chiropractors should disregard suggestions that they need lifetime care.

Whiplash Scams

Chiropractic advertisements often suggest that victims of automobile accidents can develop neck trouble years after an accident occurs. This can certainly happen when an obvious injury causes immediate neck pain. But some ads imply that neck trouble can occur years after an accident, even when there are no initial signs or symptoms of injury. Chiropractors who place these ads maintain that subluxations occur without symptoms and can start a degenerative process that becomes apparent years later. This is nonsense!

If you have a minor accident and have no neck pain or other symptoms within a few days or weeks after the accident, there is no reason to believe that an injury has occurred that will cause trouble later. Persons who get such misinformation from chiropractic advertisements will often go for a free x-ray exam months or years after an uneventful auto accident. Even though they are symptom-free, a chiropractor might tell them that they have early degenerative changes that are the result of accident-related sub-luxations and that chiropractic treatment is needed to prevent further degeneration.

Some people who are led to believe that they are developing a serious neck problem will hire an attorney. Many cases have come to light in which unethical chiropractors team up with mercenary attorneys to develop lucrative "personal injury" practice. This has become a big problem for insurance carriers and to policyholders whose premiums are raised to cover the expense of defending against unwarranted claims.

If you have an auto accident and no neck injury becomes apparent within a few days, you are very unlikely to develop accident-related symptoms years afterwards. Most people gradually develop degenerative changes as they age, but it would be incorrect to blame an accident for them—and most do not necessitate treatment.

The bottom line is that people who are not having neck pain do not need neck treatment. Remember that cervical manipulation should never be done unnecessarily. If you are feeling well, do not respond to a "free examination" offer for people who "have ever had an auto accident."

More Scare Tactics

Chiropractic advertisements often warn readers that headaches, stiff neck, insomnia, pain between the shoulder blades, painful joints, fatigue, indigestion, backache, nervousness, pain or numbness in the arms or legs, and/or various other common symptoms are "danger signals." One ad, for example, states that "these symptoms are the usual forerunner of a serious condition" and that "tension on spinal nerves robs your body of vital energy." Typically, the advertiser offers a free examination, after which the prospect is advised that chiropractic care is needed.

"Straight" chiropractic groups communicate similar messages. The Web site of the World Chiropractic Alliance (WCA), for example, states:

> It's very rare to find someone with a spine that's perfectly aligned. In most people, the spine curves slightly to the right or left and sometimes, one or more of the vertebrae are twisted or rotated.
>
> When the vertebrae are misaligned, the flow of messages from the brain to all the other cells in the body are distorted. This type of nerve interference creates dis-organization of bodily processes and dis-ease. This misalignment of the vertebrae can often exist undetected and slowly undermine one's health.

WCA, which was founded in 1989, is "dedicated to promoting a subluxation-free world" [153]. Its founder and president, Terry A. Rondberg, D.C., also created the Vertebral Subluxation Research Institute (VSRI), a now-defunct practice-building program to "stem the tide of what we call the silent killer." According to a VSRI brochure:

> *The Silent Killer* exists in the human body when the vertebrae move in and out of place and cause an interference in the nerves' ability to carry messages from the brain. Those messages are critical for optimum functioning of your body.
>
> When the vertebrae move out of place, you have what is known as a *VERTEBRAL SUBLUXATION—The Silent Killer.*

Rondberg's book *Chiropractic First* recommends "Chiropractic first, drugs second, and surgery last" and advises that spinal adjustments to remove nerve interference will help any patient who is "alive and has a nervous system." A 1992 survey of WCA members found that 81 percent thought that "killer subluxation" was an accurate term and only 15% considered it an overstatement used to frighten and mislead patients [193].

Although the "killer subluxation" notion is rarely tied to an identifiable illness, at least one chiropractor has related it to sudden death with heart disease:

> "Killer subluxation" may be a preposterous notion to the medically-minded public; it may be ridiculed by our medical counterparts as speculative and quackery; it may be embarrassing to those DC's who cannot properly explain the concept of "unbalanced activation of sympathetic nerves"; but the fact remains that "killer subluxation" may be a very real phenomenon in the role of cardiac arrest. . . . Unfortunately, most people today are unaware of the Big Idea of neuro-physiology—how the nerve system controls body functions. Although most people acknowledge chiropractic's effectiveness with back pain, most remain uninformed about the greater impact of spinal adjustments. . . .
>
> How many more people will die before they learn that chiropractic care is good for more than just back attacks? [171]

Some chiropractors claim that untreated spines often degenerate in stages, leading to disability, and that regular spinal care can prevent progression from one stage to another. Patients made fearful that their spine "is in the process of degenerating" are more receptive to "preventative-maintenance."

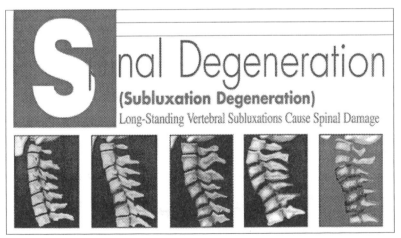

This depicts a normal spine on the left and "four states of degeneration" that some chiropractors claim will occur unless subluxations are detected and corrected in their early stages. This tactic is pure nonsense.

"Chiropractic Pediatrics"

Many chiropractors and chiropractic associations recommend spinal adjustments for infants and children [174]. The leader in this movement is the International Chiropractic Association (ICA), whose Council on Chiropractic Pediatrics offers the chiropractic profession's only "board certification" in chiropractic pediatrics. The ICA states that the council is one of its fastest-growing specialty groups [91].

Dr. Terry Rondberg's *Chiropractic First* recommends that everyone be checked for nerve interference shortly after birth and regularly throughout life. Citing a D.D. Palmer pronouncement that "Chiropractors correct abnormalities of the intellect as well as that of the body," Rondberg asserts that "chiropractic can help an average child become above average" and "perhaps a child's I.Q. can be raised—reading skills improved, etc., as well as being given an edge in alertness, coordination and speech." He recommends that "all children be checked regularly for nerve interference, even without symptoms present" and that parents be urged to consider chiropractic care if their child suffers from:

> Fever, colic, croup, allergies, wheezing, poor posture, stomach ache, hearing loss, neck/back pain, leg/hip/foot pain, numbness, headaches, coughs/colds, asthma, bed wetting, bronchitis, constipation, weakness/fatigue, ear infections, skin problems, one leg shorter, irritability, neck aches, nervousness, learning disorders, sinus problems, eye problems, scoliosis, arthritis, fatigue, pain in joints, shoulder/arm pain, poor concentration. [153]

The Singer pamphlet "Children and Chiropractic" states:

> If the human spine withstands an incredible amount of pressure from everyday activities such as twisting, turning, pulling, and lifting, imagine the stress an active, playful child can put on his spine. Children's growing, developing bodies may receive more stress in a single day than many adults receive in an entire year! It's no wonder then that a child's spine is more susceptible to injury than an adult's.... Many common childhood ailments that used to be passed off as "phases" a child goes through, or inherent in children are now being traced to spinal misalignments. Chiropractors have successfully treated colic, sleep disorders, bed wetting, constipation, allergies and asthma, scoliosis and hyperactivity....
>
> Regular chiropractic examinations are as important for your child's health as medical and dental check-ups. Early detection of misalignments can prevent permanent damage to your child's still developing systems. [170d]

Pediatric Chiropractic, a textbook published in 1998 by Williams & Wilkins, asserts that trouble begins before birth:

> The chiropractor has an opportunity to normalize, if not minimize, the effects of vertebral subluxation complex. Thorough analysis and specific adjustments to the pregnant female and pediatric spine may have a far-reaching impact on whole body health. [33]

This book alleges that the spine can be traumatized by certain positions of the fetus in the uterus, the birth process, certain diapering techniques, lifting the child from a crib or car seat, use of a baby walker, sleeping on the stomach, slumping in a chair, falls, and sports activities. The chapter on adjustment techniques occupies one hundred pages and contains more than two hundred illustrations.

A chiropractor who specializes in pediatrics and markets educational materials made this report after examining a twelve-hour-old infant:

> The newborn was analyzed for vertebral subluxations (V.S.) and general wellness. CBP® analysis was used and V.S. were found in the cervical and thoracic spines. The newborn was adjusted and placed on an intensive schedule to correct the V.S. Once normal measurements are obtained, he will be released for lifetime chiropractic wellness care. [141]

Eric Plasker, D.C., who practices in Atlanta, recently founded the Traumatic Brain Syndrome Research Foundation to investigate his contention that "traumatic birth may result in vertebral subluxation in the newborn." Plasker hopes that the foundation can establish protocols and develop research that will "attract a new level of attention to correcting vertebral subluxations in children." He also founded the Chiropractic Mothers Morning Out™ program, which uses "an army" of mothers and mothers-to-be to spread the word. According to a recent ad, his first three programs produced "46 committed, lifetime new patients and an extra $31,000." Plasker also suggests that his program can enable chiropractors to "turn every new patient you get into a Chiropractic Family for life" [144].

About five years ago, a *Consumer Reports* editor wrote to 456 chiropractors chosen randomly from the American Chiropractic Association membership directory. Posing as a prospective patient, she said she was looking for a chiropractor who could care for herself, her husband, three children, and a mother-in-law. Most of the 274 chiropractors who responded stated that they *focused* on family health care, and nearly half specifically mentioned that chiropractic can benefit children or sent booklets with that implication [37].

There are several good reasons why chiropractors should not be treating infants and children. Chiropractors do not have adequate training in the care and diagnosis of pediatric ailments, and they lack access to antibiotics and other medical treatment methods that may be needed to combat potentially fatal or crippling illnesses. Chiropractors who believe that subluxated vertebrae cause disease and that spinal adjustment is the treatment of choice are predisposed to adjusting the spine from the moment of birth. Even worse, many if not most of them are philosophically opposed to immunization.

The spine of an infant or child differs greatly from that of an adult. During the growth period, until about age twelve or thirteen, the cartilaginous growth centers of the vertebrae are soft and fragile, and the spine is very flexible. An adult whose spine stiffens or locks as a result of degenerative changes or other problems can sometimes benefit from spinal manipulation. But a small child's spine rarely, if ever, has a problem that warrants its use. There is no reason to believe that the vertebrae in the largely cartilaginous spine of an infant or toddler will bind or slip out of alignment. "Adjusting" the soft bones of infants places unnecessary strain on growth centers that form the vertebrae and on the delicate ligaments that hold them together. During my forty-three years of practice, I never manipulated an infant and only treated a few children under age twelve, all of whom had musculoskeletal problems and were referred by a pediatrician or an orthopedist.

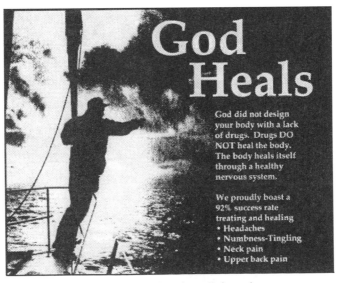

Some chiropractors invoke religious themes.

Inappropriate X-Ray Examinations

Rational chiropractors use x-ray examination only when pain and other red flags indicate a need for it. If you don't have pain, it is not likely that you need your spine x-rayed (see Chapter 6). When indicated, x-rays should focus on the spinal area where pain is present (or where referred pain originates). In the case of Susan B, who had a mechanical-type low-back pain, for example, neck x-rays should not have been taken.

Full-spine x-rays should never be used as a screening device. One full-spine x-ray (on a 14" x 36" sheet of film) exposes a person's sexual organs to between ten and one thousand times as much radiation as a chest x-ray [22]. Full-spine x-ray films lack the detail obtainable in smaller, more focused views of a problem area. Even when regional x-rays are made, the fewer the better. According to a prominent orthopedic specialist, a routine set of spinal x-rays in a young woman has a radiation effect on her ovaries equivalent to chest x-rays administered daily for sixty days! [197]

Some chiropractors advertise a free x-ray exam to determine whether chiropractic treatment is appropriate for your particular problem. You should assume that chiropractors who do this are looking for "subluxations" and will always find them and recommend treatment. The same should be assumed for chiropractors who offer screenings with thermography, contour analysis, SEMG, or the other imaging procedures described in Chapter 10. Chiropractors who offer these procedures usually want to repeat them periodically—at patient expense—which would unnecessarily raise the cost of their care. The most prudent consumer action is to ignore all offers of free chiropractic examinations and to avoid chiropractors who offer them.

Claims Galore

Another promotional strategy is to suggest that chiropractic's scope is unlimited. Many chiropractors display charts and brochures depicting connections between spinal segments and body organs. Some associate the spinal levels with various organs (see page 42), while others list specific conditions (see pages 6 and 41). Although spinal nerves contain some fibers connecting to autonomic nerves that supply the viscera, no single spinal nerve controls the function of an internal organ—and even if one did, there is no reason to believe that spinal manipulation would influence any such function. Chiropractors who limit their practice to treating back pain and other musculoskeletal problems do not use such charts.

Peter G. Fernandez, D.C., practice-building consultant and author *of 1001 Ways to Attract New Patients* and *How to Become a Million Dollar a Year Practitioner,* advises chiropractors:

Learn how to fix all varieties of headaches, internal problems, pediatric ailments, health problems of the elderly, nutritional problems, etc. . . .

Many other practitioners will state, because of their lack of training, experience, or philosophy, that chiropractic can't fix colitis, ulcers, kidney problems, hormonal imbalances, etc. To those doctors who feel this way, I encourage you to take postgraduate instruction on these problems. You will be surprised. Chiropractic works a lot better than you think it will. My experience as a chiropractor is: "Two of my patients that were blind, now see; two people who were deaf, now hear; and many people who were lame . . . now walk." I've cured epilepsy, liver problems, gall bladder problems, *etc., etc.* Please don't misinterpret my comments as egocentric. I'm not. I didn't actually cure these people. All I did was find the subluxations, reduce them, keep them reduced, and the patient's bodies healed. The point I am trying to make is CHIROPRACTIC WORKS. When you expand the variety of conditions you treat, your practice will increase. [59]

In 1998, a Hawaiian chiropractor distributed flyers claiming that "chiropractic healing successfully treats" cancer, epilepsy, leukemia, and more than sixty other conditions. Although such flamboyance is rare, the situation has special significance because a supervising investigator for the state licensing board issued this response to a complaint:

This case has been inactivated with a disposition of "No Violation." Evidence submitted was reviewed by a licensed chiropractor serving as a member of the Advisory Committee of the Chiropractic Board of our department.

Thousands of chiropractors have misleading literature in their offices. During the past several years, the most prolific publisher has been Tedd Koren, D.C., of Philadelphia, doing business as Koren Publications. During 1998, Koren's fifty-four pamphlets included: "Allergies," "Are You Popping Pills?" "Asthma & Emphysema," "Blood Pressure," "Ear Infections," "Healthier Children with Chiropractic," "Infants & Babies," "Strengthen Your Immune System," and "Why Should I Return If I'm Feeling Fine?" His *Chiropractic: Bringing Out the Best In You* booklet includes fever, croup, bedwetting, ear infections, sore throat, eye problems, cough, asthma, bronchitis, poor concentration, and thirty-four other problems on a "partial list" of childhood conditions within chiropractic's scope [110]. Koren also advises chiropractors they can double their practice "practically overnight" by having patients read the list and asking: "Do you know of any children, perhaps your own, or those of relatives or friends, that have any of the problems in this list?" [112]

The Federal Trade Commission (FTC) appears to be concerned about Koren's claims. Although the agency does not publicly discuss pending actions, Koren himself has provided many of the details. According to an article in *Dynamic Chiropractic*, FTC attorneys want to prohibit him from making any unsubstantiated claim that chiropractic: (a) improves human immunocompetence; (b) reduces the incidence in children of ear infection, allergies, or tonsillitis; (c) administered to children is effective in the treatment or amelioration of asthma, anxiety, low-mental stamina, inability to concentrate, hyperactivity, discipline problems, low grades, or low IQ; (d) is comparable or superior in effectiveness to vaccinations as a means of preventing common childhood diseases, including measles, mumps, German measles, and chicken pox; and (e) administered to children increases their resistance to common childhood diseases, including measles, mumps, German measles, and chicken pox. The FTC's proposed agreement would also prohibit any unsubstantiated representation "about the health benefits,

---

Sparrow & Jacobs, Colorado Springs, Colorado markets greeting cards. The cover of its Fall/Holiday 1998 catalog states, " Increase your patient traffic! . . . If you don't market to your patients, other doctors will!" Various cards state:

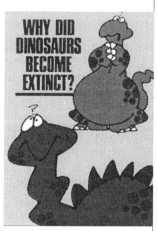

- All stressed out and nowhere to go? Try Chiropractic! It's the natural way to relieve the toll stress can take on your health and peace of mind. Call us today for an appointment!
- Chiropractic is nature's answer toward the changing tides of life. Take the first step toward natural stress relief by giving us a call!
- The first step toward awakening your body's natural healing process is giving us a call. Let us help you feel your very best.
- Chiropractic's gentle healing brings you back into nature's balance.
- Chiropractic is a natural way to release the tensions of modern life and nurture the benefits of better health.
- Why did dinosaurs become extinct? They failed to adjust! Thanks to chiropractic, you should be around for a long time! [birthday message]
- Why did dinosaurs become extinct? Because they never helped their kids adjust! But YOU can, with kid-friendly Chiropractic care!

performance, or efficacy of chiropractic, or any substantially similar treatment" [62].

Chiropractic's most widely distributed patient-education booklet is *Introduction to Chiropractic: A Natural Method of Health Care*, by Louis Sportelli, D.C. Sportelli, a former chairman of the American Chiropractic Association's board of governors, reflects the "mixer" viewpoint. While specifying no diseases, he asserts:

> Locating minor spinal deviations early, before they interfere with a proper functioning nervous system and produce symptoms, will greatly assist your body in remaining healthy. . . .
> Regular spinal adjustments are a part of your body's defense against illness. . . .
> The conditions which doctors of chiropractic treat can be as varied and as vast as the nervous system itself. [180]

A California chiropractor is offering free e-mail consultations based on a questionnaire posted on her Web site. The questionnaire, adapted from the nerve chart pictured on page 41, lists "areas controlled by nerves" and "possible effects of a malfunction." The "possible effects" include crossed eyes, liver conditions, sore throat, sterility, thyroid conditions, whooping cough, and approximately one hundred other diseases and conditions, very few of which have any relevance to chiropractic care [45].

LK Graphic Communications, of Belle Vernon, Pennsylvania, distributes Singer pamphlets, and many other subluxation-based educational materials. One is a series of newsletters relating chiropractic care to allergies, arthritis, the immune system, heart disease, and general health. The "Heart Wise" issue advises readers to "protect your heart" by eating right, exercising, stopping smoking, and "keeping it in balance with chiropractic." An accompanying photo shows a woman getting her neck adjusted.

Of course, claims can also be made vaguely. The Alliance for Chiropractic Progress, a partnership of the American Chiropractic Association, the International Chiropractors Association, and the Association of Chiropractic Colleges, is advertising that "as more and more people realize the scope of what chiropractic can do for whole body healing and health maintenance, they are turning to a doctor of chiropractic to treat more conditions—with great success." The ads also suggest that medical care is unwarranted unless chiropractic care fails [4]. The Alliance's ultimate goal is to position chiropractors as "highly trained and qualified health care providers who offer consumers a credible choice in providing health care for their families" [3].

Education or Brainwashing?

Practice-building programs are literally designed to *create* chiropractic patients and to recruit entire families into lifetime care. Without patients who are totally committed to "maintenance care," it may take years to build a properly limited practice that is respected by consumers and healthcare professionals alike.

Practice-building experts present "patient education" as the key to helping suffering humanity and building a lucrative practice. Dennis Nikitow, founder of The Ca$h Practice Seminar, states that patients who understand subluxation concepts will usually include chiropractic in their health care [132]. In a recent issue of the International Chiropractic Association's journal, he explained:

> The truth in practicing chiropractic lies in the philosophy. It is the core of the "traditional" chiropractors' beliefs and the "way" behind their practice. The simplicity of it is, chiropractors adjust the spine to maximize nerve integrity, improve body function and increase health potential. When patients understand this, several things happen:
>
> 1. They see chiropractic as something they need to do for health, not for pain.
> 2. They begin maintaining their spine through regular adjustments.
> 3. They bring their families in to maintain their spines.
> 4. They put a chiropractor on their health care team.
> 5. They pay for care regardless of insurance reimbursement.
> 6. They educate and refer others who are just treating their symptoms.

Chiropractic newspapers are filled with ads for seminars, reports, and practice-building aids headlined with promises of financial success. For example:

> GET RICH . . . Play this exciting 30-minute infomercial and get over 1000 new patients!
> Double Your Practice in 24 Months or Less!
> The Lazy Doctor Way To Make $20,000 a Week, Using Little Known Secrets For Getting Personal Injury Patients!
> You Will Laugh at Money Worries – with a MD/DC/PT Rehab Clinic! Business income secrets revealed . . .
> Imagine What Your Life Could Be Like With 10-20 New Personal Injury Cases Per Month!
> EARN AN *EXTRA* $50,000 *MINIMUM* IN YOUR PRACTICE IN THE NEXT 12 MONTHS—*GUARANTEED!*

How a small town Pennsylvania Chiropractor went from embarrassed and broke to attracting patients *in just 3 weeks* and generating over 92,338 visits *in 48 months*.
Want more cash-paying, highly motivated patients?

Stephen Barrett, M.D., has analyzed instructional materials from more than a dozen chiropractic practice-builders and found that nearly all include tips on selling lifetime maintenance care. The most explicit presentation is the 238-page *Dynamic Essentials Seminars Procedures Manual*, written by Life University president Sid E. Williams, D.C. This book, the first edition of which was published about thirty years ago, provides responses to nearly every conceivable objection to periodic checkups and adjustments [199].

Williams divides the initial phase of patient contact into three parts: the consultation, the examination (including an x-ray examination of every patient), and the report of findings. Page 26 states:

> The examination procedures are more than diagnostic, they are to emphasize to the patient that a weakness exists in his body and that it has been caused by spinal fixations. By fortifying the patient's knowledge of the "spinal cause" by the use of test instruments and graphs, the patient is able to see beyond any doubt that he is actually physically sick, that a spinal condition caused it, and that something needs to be done chiropractically to correct it.

Williams recommends that after the initial symptoms are relieved, the patient should be persuaded to continue monthly "preventive maintenance." (Page 52 notes that "A very excellent doctor-patient relationship can be built up once the patient has experienced relief through chiropractic adjustments, and he will accept almost any reasonable recommendation of time – correction.") If the patient asks, "But will I have to continue with chiropractic care as long as I live?" the recommended reply (page 104) is:

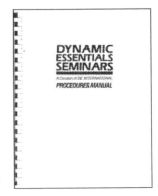

> (Chuckling) No ma'am, you won't have to continue it as long as you live. Only as long as you want to stay healthy. (Pause) Every spine needs some maintenance, Mrs. Jones. My family and I are checked regularly on a monthly basis, and more often when we think that it is necessary. Yes, if you want to stay healthy, you will have to continue some chiropractic care.

Pages 145–149 describe a technique called "sealing the patient in." First the patient is asked if various positive responses have occurred "yet." If any have, he is told he even looks better. Then he is instructed to rest quietly in the chiropractor's office so he can get "filled up with the thought that he is better, looks better, and he will be able to tell all his friends how much better he is." But page 149 warns:

> Keep in mind that we don't want to feature "Well" or "Cure" too soon or too strongly because the patient won't show up for the next visit since he thinks "I'm ready to quit; I am well." Remember, most patients have been locked in to the medical perspective of "curing" disease. Once a "cure" is achieved, medical care is terminated.
>
> Don't emphasize improvement too fast. Instead we say, "We want to get you over on the good side of the ledger and keep you there."

The American Chiropractic Association's book *Developing a Chiropractic Practice* suggests adopting a philosophy that "enters into and colors all financial, administrative, clinical, and human relations functions of the practice." When sound office philosophy is expressed, the book says, "the doctor and assistants will just naturally do and say things" that will promote referrals. For example, they will:

1. Impress your patients with the results they have realized.
2. Take the initiative to suggest chiropractic health care when anyone mentions a sick or disabled friend or relative.
3. Have a system of motivational communications.
4. Suggest to patients that they mention chiropractic to friends, relatives, neighbors, and associates when patients are at the peak of their enthusiasm.

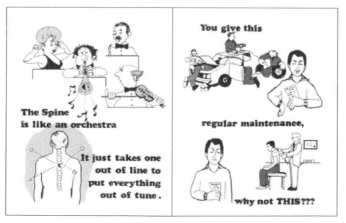

Many chiropractors use simple analogies to promote their services [143].

5. Patronize worthy patients who are attorneys, dentists, optometrists, druggists, retailers, insurance agents, contractors, etc., even if you can get the same products or services slightly cheaper at another location. [160]

Back Talk Systems, which markets an extensive line of motivational products, calls referrals "the ultimate compliment." One of its flyers advises patients that "the best way to thank your doctor is to tell others" [151].

Indoctrinating Employees

Many chiropractors train their receptionists and office employees to promote chiropractic and to solicit patients. It is a common practice for such chiropractors to take their "office girls" to practice-building seminars where they are indoctrinated in chiropractic philosophy and taught to believe that chiropractic is a superior method of healing. In order to facilitate such brainwashing, chiropractors often hire employees who "believe in chiropractic" because of previous experience they have had with chiropractors. Noting that "you cannot sell a product in which you do not believe," Share International, the largest practice-building organization, has advised:

> The best receptionist is usually one who has been a chiropractic patient FIRST. . . .
> Give your receptionist regular adjustments. Impress her from the beginning that she represents chiropractic in your office. She MUST look and feel healthy if she is going to sell "health" to your patients. Give her an adjustment for a cold, for cramps, for a headache, until she actually realizes for herself, "Say, this REALLY DOES work!!" Then when she is asked if chiropractic works for a certain condition, she BELIEVES in the product she is selling. [68]

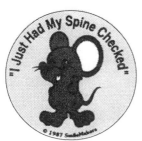 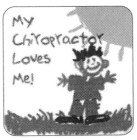 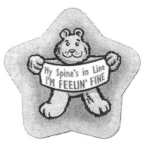

Stickers, refrigerator magnets, bookmarks, bent ("subluxated") pens, key rings, mugs, coloring books, T-shirts, calendars, postcards, and other novelty items may be used to reinforce the "maintenance" care message.

Not long ago, a niece of mine who lives in Alabama applied for a position as a receptionist in a chiropractic office and was immediately hired when she stated that her grandfather and her uncle were chiropractors. When she called to tell me that she had been hired, I warned that the chiropractor might attempt to use her to build his practice by having her talk patients into returning for treatment they did not need. Her indoctrination began with a practice-building seminar in Orlando, Florida, where she was told that chiropractic could cure or prevent most ailments and that it was her moral duty to encourage patients and their children to return for ongoing chiropractic care. My niece had a six-month-old baby girl. I told her that under no circumstances should she let the chiropractor treat her baby. When her baby developed a 102°F fever, the chiropractor offered treatment. He also advised against vaccination. When my niece refused to follow his advice and instead took her baby to a pediatrician, the chiropractor pressured her into quitting since "she did not fit in."

"You were right," my niece told me later. "The chiropractor tried to make me believe that medical care was dangerous and ineffective. After you warned me, I was able to see that he was trying to brainwash me." I'm sure the chiropractor was surprised to find that the niece of a chiropractor did not "believe in chiropractic." It is unfortunate that many unsuspecting employees of chiropractors are subjected to instruction that requires total devotion to the chiropractor's particular brand of healing.

Advance Payments

Some chiropractors offer a discount if payment is made in advance for a series of treatments. The patient might then be set up on a schedule of daily visits for a few weeks, every-other-day visits for a few months, and then bimonthly visits that are gradually reduced to monthly visits for the rest of the patient's lifetime. Some chiropractors require that the patient sign an agreement to undergo a certain number of treatments "so that the treatment will be more effective."

Although some chiropractors believe so strongly in the vertebral subluxation theory that they honestly feel that regular spinal adjustments should be a part of your disease-prevention program, prepayment treatment plans and "preventative-maintenance" spinal adjustments are more often for the benefit of the chiropractor than the patient.

It is difficult or impossible to determine beforehand how many treatments a patient might need. Neck or back pain that has been present for only a few days will often be relieved with two or three treatments or will spontaneously resolve after four or five days, making further treatment unnecessary. A simple neck crick (muscle spasm) that occasionally greets people when they awaken in the morning may disappear within a few days. A simple back strain usually resolves in less than two weeks. Pain that persists longer than four weeks may need a special examination or a different treatment method.

Chiropractors who encourage advance payment for a long course of spinal adjustments generally will continue adjusting imaginary subluxations long after the patient's symptoms have disappeared. I usually advise my patients to go by how they feel and stop treatment when they feel okay. If treatment aggravates their pain, or if symptoms have not subsided after a few weeks, a different treatment or a different doctor might be indicated.

Obviously, it would be unwise to pay in advance for a long course of treatments if there is a chance that you might need only a few treatments or if there is a question about the diagnosis. Unnecessary spinal manipulation could pose an unnecessary risk, especially with neck manipulation.

Prepayment treatment plans are often recommended by practice-building advisers and are a big problem in the chiropractic profession, especially when they involve requests for reimbursement from insurance carriers. Because insurance companies and HMOs generally refuse to pay for "maintenance care," some chiropractors are taking courses in how to run a "cash practice." Chiropractors must convince patients that the treatment they offer is so essential for good health that the patient will be willing to "prepay in full" without involving an insurance carrier. It is never a good idea to pay for chiropractic treatments in advance.

Don't Get Oversold

An appropriate program of hands-on manipulation, physical therapy measures, rest, and/or exercise may relieve symptoms or speed recovery. Even without treatment, 70 percent of patients with acute back pain will recover in three weeks, 90 percent in two months. When people feel better after receiving treatment, they are apt to trust whatever explanation they receive about their problem.

My advice is simple: If you encounter talk of subluxations, abnormal curvatures, preventative maintenance, or any of the other sales tactics described in this chapter, either ignore them or go elsewhere. If you stay, make sure that any manipulative treatment you undergo is near the area of pain rather than at a remote area. And when you feel better, stop going.

9

Nutrition
Nonsense

Chiropractic surveys suggest that at least 80 percent of chiropractors are giving nutrition advice to their patients [38,87]. As far as I can tell, the nature of this advice has not been systematically tabulated. Some chiropractors are able to counsel their patients about sensible eating, weight control, and other nutrition-related health matters. Many, however, are engaged in questionable nutrition practices.

All chiropractic colleges teach courses in basic and clinical nutrition. Although most courses rely on standard nutrition textbooks, it is not clear whether students put what they learn to good use. Practicing chiropractors have little exposure to science-based nutrition. Chiropractic journals, magazines, and textbooks provide very little nutrition information, and most of what they provide is not valid. Postgraduate seminars are available, but the vast majority are sponsored by supplement distributors for the purpose of boosting sales. During my forty-three-year career, I have seen hundreds of advertisements for such seminars. I cannot recall a single one that appeared to provide valid teachings. Many state chiropractic associations promote similarly questionable seminars that yield credits toward license renewal. Many exhibitors at chiropractic conventions hawk supplements that are sold in chiropractic offices. Some exhibitors promote inappropriate diagnostic tests, and some even distribute literature stating which products supposedly are effective against various diseases.

Chiropractors interested in science-based nutrition can pick up the basics from other sources or by studying on their own. It is not difficult to learn enough to answer the questions patients typically ask about food composition, dietary balance, osteoporosis prevention, exercise principles, low-fat eating, and other dietary strategies. However, many chiropractors mix nutrition and subluxation theory, use dubious tests, or engage in bizarre treatment systems that result in inappropriate use of supplement products. This chapter will help you judge the validity of nutrition-related practices you may encounter in a chiropractic office.

Supplement Promotion

Chiropractors can greatly augment their income by selling nutritional products to their patients. More than fifty companies market them primarily or exclusively through chiropractors. Some handle just a few products, while others sell hundreds. These products are typically sold for two to three times what the chiropractor pays for them. Various tests may be used to persuade patients to buy them.

• Functional Intracellular Analysis (FIA), formerly called Essential Metabolics Analysis (EMA), is a test in which a sample of the patient's blood is sent to a laboratory that isolates the patient's lymphocytes (a type of white blood cell) and places them into petri dishes containing various concentrations of certain nutrients. Company literature states that the procedure can find hidden "functional" nutrient deficiencies in nearly everyone. Although properly performed lymphocyte cultures have a legitimate role in testing for certain deficiencies, they are not appropriate for screening as advocated by the laboratory [24].

• Hair analysis is done by clipping a sample of the patient's hair—usually from the nape of the neck—and sending it to a laboratory for analysis. The lab then issues a report (often with a copy for the patient) stating the concentrations of various minerals and how these amounts compare to the lab's reference values. Some reports also contain specific recommendations for supplements. The scientific viewpoint is that hair tests of this sort do not provide a valid basis for determining the body's nutritional state or for making supplement recommendations [18,72].

• Live blood analysis—also called live cell analysis, nutritional blood analysis, and Hemaview—is done by placing a drop of the patient's blood on a microscope slide and using a glass cover slip to keep it from drying out. The slide is then viewed with a special microscope that forwards the image to a television monitor that the practitioner and patient can view. Although certain blood characteristics (such as the relative size of the red cells) are visible with this setup, live-cell analysts invariably misinterpret other things, such as the extent of red blood cell clumping and changes in the shape of the cells that occur as the blood sample dries. The results are then used as a basis for prescribing supplements. Chiropractors using this approach typically advise patients to take vitamins and/or enzyme pills and to return periodically for checkups. The Web site of one imaginative chiropractor advises that, "By checking the blood, we check the oil of the body. It can tell us a great deal about the body, and whether or not it is able to keep up with the stress of everyday life, or if it is on its way to problems down the road."

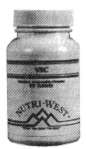
A product "formulated . . . specifically for Subluxation based practices." Such products are typically claimed to help "hold" vertebrae in place after an adjustment.

• "Nutrient deficiency" questionnaires typically contain a long list of symptoms and conditions that the patient checks off. The information is then fed into a computer that reports what products the patient should take. Some symptoms might occur in a vitamin deficiency disease or glandular disorder, but many have nothing to do with nutritional status. The questionnaire might also ask about diet, health habits, or other lifestyle factors. The computers are programmed to recommend products for everyone.

Dubious Treatment Systems

Many chiropractors use elaborate systems that include a nutrition component. The numbers using such systems range from a few hundred to many thousands.

• Applied kinesiology (AK) is based on the idea that every organ dysfunction is accompanied by a specific muscle weakness, which enables health problems to be diagnosed through muscle-testing procedures. Testing is typically carried out by pulling on the patient's outstretched arm. Proponents claim that nutritional deficiencies, allergies, and other adverse reactions to foods or nutrients can be detected by having the patient chew or suck on them or by placing them on the tongue so that the patient salivates. Some practitioners have the test material held in the patient's hand or placed on another part of the body. A few even perform "surrogate testing" in which the arm strength of a parent is tested to diagnose problems in a child held by the parent. Many muscle-testing proponents assert that nutrients tested in these various ways will have an immediate effect, that "good" substances will strengthen specific muscles, whereas "bad" substances will cause weaknesses that indicate trouble with the associated organ or tissue. The recommended "treatment" can include special diets, food supplements, acupressure, and spinal manipulation. A 1991 survey by the National Board of Chiropractic Examiners found that 37.2 percent of those who responded said they were practicing AK.

Some experiments with muscle-testing procedures have found no difference in muscle response from one substance to another, while others have found no difference between test substances and placebos. The International College of Applied Kinesiology (ICAK) maintains that practitioners who do not follow its standards are not doing AK, and that muscle-testing results should be combined with other clinical findings and not be used by themselves [90]. However, critics respond that the nutrition-related claims and practices of those affiliated with ICAK are no less bizarre than those of other muscle-testers who do not [17].

• Biological Terrain Assessment (BTA) uses a computerized analysis of blood, urine, and saliva specimens to recommend nutritional programs, vitamin and mineral supplements, homeopathic products, and/or herbs. Proponents claim that BTA gives evidence of disease at cellular level which enables "imbalances" to be detected and corrected in their early stages. Neither the rationale nor the recommended strategies make sense.

• Biomagnetic Therapy is based on the idea that disease cannot exist when the body is "biomagnetically balanced" and "all nutrition" is available. It has been promoted through seminars at which chiropractors are taught how to use magnetic and nutritional procedures for "normalizing organs and systems."

• Contact Reflex Analysis (CRA), an AK offshoot, involves pushing down on the patient's outstretched arm while touching "reflex points" located in various parts of the body. In a recent report, CRA developer Dick A. Versendaal, D.C., stated:

> On a healthy body, electricity flows to every area and feeds it the energy it needs to function. When you use CRA to test the reflexes of each area, the testing arm, which is like a circuit breaker, will remain strong if there is no interruption of nerve energy. However, if one area of the body has become unhealthy, it begins to draw excessive electrical energy in order to stay alive and functioning. This causes the body's electrical system to "blow a breaker": the muscle being used to perform the test (usually the deltoid muscle of the left or right arm) will become weak and the arm will drop when the affected arm reflex is tested. [190]

Proponents further claim that "weakness" of the arm points to problems in corresponding areas and that nutritional supplementation can solve these problems. A recent flyer from Parker College of Chiropractic for one-day training sessions in "Contact Reflex Analysis and Designed Clinical Nutrition" advised chiropractors that they would learn to:

• Completely examine a patient using this new method
• Find the Cause of the problem
• Prove to the patient that you have *Found the Cause*
• Show the patient that you have *Corrected the Cause*
• Demonstrate to the patient that he/she requires specific nutrients
• Simplify test procedures for Blood Pressure Syndromes and Fluid Retention
• Develop a strong analytical and nutritional alternative to medical diagnosis and drugs
• *Use a new easy* test and correction for Slipped and Ruptured disk

- Use a new test to determine nutritional needs to balance skeletal muscles, tendons, and ligaments
- Simplify procedures to test for allergies as well as nutritional alternatives to drugs
- Simplify testing procedures to determine subluxations of vertebra, spinal disks, and joints
- Use a newly revised and up-to-date textbook fully illustrated for immediate identification of the body's contact points. The index contains *1,500 conditions with nutritional protocols* to enhance patient management skills
- Use a Philosophy and a Technique that bring science and intuition into powerful focus through a dynamic healing art, uncovering a client's nutritional needs. [46]

You might think that such an all-inclusive pseudoscientific approach to diagnosis and treatment would be rejected by any member of the healing arts and would not be worthy of discussion. But this course in Contact Reflex Analysis was "proudly presented" by Parker's Postgraduate Division and the Florida Chiropractic Association as acceptable for twelve hours of the continuing education credits that some states require for license renewal.

- The Enzyme Replacement System is based on identifying and treating "enzyme deficiency states." Its developer, Howard F. Loomis, D.C., gives seminars sponsored by National College of Chiropractic and markets products "targeted to organs stressed by subluxation." The alleged deficiency states are identified by taking a history, examining the patients, obtaining a "24-hour urinalysis, " and correlating this information with "recurring spinal subluxation patterns." According to Loomis:

> With this information, a chiropractor can now become . . . the preeminent diagnostician in the healing arts today. No longer constrained in relieving symptomatic complaints, he or she can now accurately determine the cause of non-traumatic conditions. In my experience this ability is the greatest practice-builder a doctor can possibly have. [118]

The products listed in Loomis's 1995 catalog include *Chiro-Zyme*, a line of "carefully formulated combinations of herbs, vitamins and minerals with plant enzymes," each of which is named with an abbreviation for certain spinal segments and an organ or body function. The product *C8 to T1 Thy*, for example, is claimed to "nourish the tissues of the thyroid gland stressed by subluxations of the upper thoracic and cervical spine."

• Iridology, also called iris diagnosis, maintains that each area of the body is represented by a corresponding area in the iris of the eye (the colored area around the pupil) and that the body's state of health and disease can be diagnosed from the color, texture, and location of pigment flecks in the eye. The leading proponent, Bernard Jensen, D.C., has written that "Nature has provided us with a miniature television screen showing the most remote portions of the body by way of nerve reflex responses" [96]. Iridology practitioners claim to diagnose "imbalances" that can be treated with vitamins, minerals, herbs, and similar products. Some also claim that the eye markings can reveal a complete history of past illnesses as well as previous treatment. Several well-designed studies have found that iridology practitioners who examined the same patients (or photographs of their eyes) disagreed among themselves and were unable to state what was medically wrong with the patients [40,108,169].

• The Morter HealthSystem, described in its literature as "a complete alternative healthcare system," combines Bio Energetic Synchronization Technique (B.E.S.T.) and nutritional supplementation. B.E.S.T. is based on the notion that development and repair of the body is controlled by its electromagnetic field. Advocates claim that electromagnetic imbalance causes unequal leg length, which the chiropractor can instantly correct by infusing his own electromagnetic energy at "contact points" on the patient's body until "pulsation" is felt and the patient's legs test equally long. The nutritional component includes supplements that supposedly "alkalize" the body. Proponents recommend lifelong testing and treatment beginning early in infancy.

• NutraBalance is one of several systems in which the results of legitimate blood and urine tests are fed into a computer which determines alleged "metabolic types," lists supposed problem areas, and recommends dietary changes and food supplements from a manufacturer chosen by the chiropractor. Neither the existence of the types nor the recommended nutritional strategies have been substantiated.

• Neuro Emotional Technique (NET) focuses on "releasing patients' emotional blocks stored in the body's memory." Its proponents claim that everyone has such blocks and that the body "replays" these old memories, which can adversely affect health [34]. The practitioner then uses muscle-testing (applied kinesiology) to "isolate a troublesome event" and asks the patient to hold in mind a "snapshot" of the emotional state while the chiropractor adjusts the patient's spine and acupuncture points and pre-scribes supplement products and homeopathic remedies.

• NUTRI-SPEC testing is performed by measuring the patient's breathing rate, blood pressure, body temperature, pulse, breath-holding ability, blood pressure, pupil size, tongue thickness or coating, several characteristics of the patient's saliva and urine, abdominal reflexes, and certain other reflexes. NUTRI-SPEC's scoring system is then used to determine whether the patient is in or out of "water/electrolyte balance," "anaerobic/dysaerobic balance," "acid/alkaline balance," and "sympathetic/parasympathetic balance" and whether the patient has "sex hormone insufficiency," "myocardial insufficiency," "pineal stress," "thymus stress," or another fanciful condition. The findings are then used to recommend dietary changes and supplements that are purchasable from the company marketing the system. The procedures are described in detail in a videotape and large manual distributed by NUTRI-SPEC's chief proponent [166].

"Cookbook" Approaches

Many supplement manufacturers offer nutritional products intended for the treatment of disease. The majority of these products do not work and are not legal to market for this purpose. In addition, many are marketed for conditions that chiropractors are not trained to diagnose or treat. Instead of making therapeutic claims openly, the manufacturers market through distributors who make the claims for them by sponsoring seminars at which speakers describe how to use the products. Some distributors give out manuals listing which products to use for which diseases. The extent to which this clandestine activity takes place is unknown.

This sixty-page booklet was published by a chiropractor in 1989. One section lists products "recommended to provide nutritional support" for adrenal gland weakness, bronchitis, emphysema, epilepsy, glaucoma, kidney stones, pinworms, pneumonia, swallowing difficulty, and about forty other conditions, most of which are far outside the scope of rational chiropractic practice. The booklet also tabulates the products of two manufacturers and their suggested uses. The author states that the information was "compiled from specific recommendations made by various manufacturers" and is intended "for information purposes only." [198]

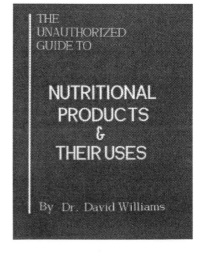

THE
UNAUTHORIZED
GUIDE TO

NUTRITIONAL
PRODUCTS
&
THEIR USES

By Dr. David Williams

Some manufacturers sell "glandular" products containing small amounts of freeze-dried animal tissue claimed to strengthen or rejuvenate the corresponding parts of the user's body. Such claims make about as much sense as the primitive notion that eating the heart of a lion will make you courageous. "Glandular" products are not legally permitted to contain hormones. Like plant-based oral enzyme products, their main ingredients are proteins that are broken down during digestion and exert no significant effect on body function.

Questionable Food Allergies

Some chiropractors use various test procedures that supposedly determine "hidden allergies" responsible for a broad range of diseases or symptoms. The most notorious of these was cytotoxic testing, which was performed by observing what happens to the patient's white blood cells after they are placed onto slides containing dried foods. Cytotoxic testing was banned by the FDA, but other tests are used for the same purpose. The most notable of these are ELISA/ACT and ALCAT testing. Some chiropractors claim that they can diagnose food allergies through electrodermal testing, a procedure described in Chapter 12.

Multilevel Products

Many chiropractors become distributors for multilevel companies that sell supplements, herbs, and/or homeopathic products. Multilevel marketing (MLM) is a form of direct sales in which "independent distributors" can buy products "wholesale," sell them "retail," and recruit other distributors who can do the same. When enough distributors have been enrolled, the recruiter is eligible to collect a percentage of their sales. During the past twenty years, Dr. Stephen Barrett has investigated over a hundred health-related MLM companies and found that every one of them has marketed products that were overpriced, misrepresented, or both.

Actual and Potential Harm

Most of the practices described above are used to varying degrees by offbeat medical doctors, dentists, naturopaths, acupuncturists, and various other practitioners who consider themselves qualified to do "nutrition counseling." However, the number of chiropractors using them appears to be much higher than that of any other practitioner type.

Although no statistics indicate how much harm is associated with these practices, there is good reason to believe it is considerable. Most of the harm is economic. Supplements sold through chiropractic offices tend to be expensive, and some are recommended for lifelong use. Psychologic harm occurs when healthy people are persuaded that they are ill. To this must be added the cost of unnecessary medical diagnostic procedures required to reassure patients that they do not have the diseases suggested by dubious tests. It also seems probable that chiropractors who think nonsensically about nutrition may be prone to other errors of professional judgment.

Physical harm, although uncommon, can occur when excessive dosages are prescribed. In 1992, a fifty-year-old Pennsylvania woman, in apparently good health, was treated by a chiropractor for hip and leg pain resulting from an automobile accident. When the pain resolved, she told the chiropractor that she felt no further need for treatment. The chiropractor, who practiced Contact Reflex Analysis, then checked her "thyroid reflex," said the woman had a "thyroid problem," and recommended dietary supplements that contained significant amounts of iodine. The standard way to diagnose a thyroid problem is to take a medical history, perform an examination of the neck while the patient swallows, and order laboratory tests, but the chiropractor did none of these. The pills he prescribed contained more than ten times the Recommended Dietary Allowance of iodine. Within three months, they stimulated the woman's thyroid gland to produce excessive amounts of thyroid hormone, which triggered weight loss, severe diarrhea, and other symptoms of thyroid toxicity. The iodine also triggered Graves disease, a thyroid condition in which the eyeballs bulge. Despite medical treatment, her eyeballs swelled enough to crush the optic nerves, which caused her to become legally blind.

Although some chiropractors give rational nutrition advice to their patients, it is clear that a substantial percentage of them do not. Despite their senselessness, nearly all of the approaches described in this chapter have been promoted by articles or advertisements in chiropractic publications, and a few have been promoted through chiropractic schools and organizations. They are very much a part of the chiropractic marketplace and have been subjected to little or no criticism by their colleagues or by professional organizations. In fact, some chiropractic organizations and publications encourage their use suggesting that chiropractors are qualified to diagnose and treat a broad spectrum of disease.

10

Gadgets and
Gimmicks

Chiropractors seem to have a propensity for incorporating gadgetry into their practice. In the 1920s, Albert Abrams, M.D.—whom the AMA later dubbed "dean of gadget quacks"—invented a system of diagnosis and healing he called "Radionics." Soon more than three thousand practitioners, mainly chiropractors, were sending dried blood specimens from patients to be inserted in Abrams's "Radioscope." The diagnosis would come back on a postcard, with recommended dial settings for treatment with other Abrams machines. One of his imitators, Ruth Drown, D.C., had a long and lucrative career using the Drown Radiotherapeutic Instrument, a little black box claimed to be able to "tune in" specific organs of the body and treat a patient by remote control anywhere in the world.

During the 1950s and 1960s, several thousand chiropractors purchased "Micro-Dynameters." These devices, invented by an engineer named F.C Ellis, were claimed to be effective for diagnosing and treating the gamut of diseases. An Ellis Research Laboratories brochure stated:

> By the use of the Micro-Dynameter you can, in a few minutes, make a complete analysis of the spine for the location of nerve interference. The Micro-Dynameter will faithfully point to the major subluxation, whether it be an acute or a chronic lesion. It will take the guess work out of your practice; it will make you a true scientist; it will make you a proud chiropractor. . . .
>
> The Micro-Dynameter will also point to local infections as in teeth, sinuses, or over abdominal viscera; it will give the true picture and the exact location of the disease focus. . . .

> After an adjustic thrust has been given, a post-check can be
> made to see whether or not a correction has been made. [121]

The elaborate-looking apparatus included a meter, half a dozen dials for the
operator to adjust, and electrodes that could be applied to different areas of
the patient's body. The working component was simply a galvanometer that
reacted to skin moistness.

The Toftness Radiation Detector, marketed during the 1970s and
early 1980s, was a handheld cylindrical instrument that contained six
plastic lenses. Its inventor, Irwing N. Toftness, D.C., claimed that: (a)
compressed spinal nerves emitted electromagnetic radiation with a frequency of 69.5 gigahertz; (b) the lenses focused this energy onto a detection
plate at the top of the device; and (c) the operator could sense the radiation
level by rubbing the plate and feeling resistance to the movement of the
fingers. The purported neurologic disturbances would then be treated by
spinal adjustments. Yale University's Edmund S. Crelin, Ph.D., who tested
the device for the FDA, pointed out that radiation at 69.5 gigahertz would
penetrate only about one millimeter of body tissue, while the spinal nerves
are two to three inches from the body's surface. So even if an ailing nerve
could radiate the tiny amount of energy as claimed, the energy would be
absorbed by surrounding tissues and would not be detectable at or above the
skin [52]. About seven hundred of the devices were leased ($700 for the first
year and $100 per year for fourteen more years) to chiropractors who
completed Toftness's training course.

In each of the above situations, the FDA obtained a court order
banning further sale or distribution of the devices. As far as I know, they are
no longer being used. However, new forms of gadgets and gimmicks have
taken their place. This chapter describes several that are purported to detect
"subluxations," treat them, and/or monitor patient progress.

Activator Methods (AM)

Activator Methods Chiropractic Technique is a diagnostic and treatment
system centered on the idea that leg-length analysis can determine when to
adjust and when not to adjust the spine. Proponents claim that its procedures
"generally enable the clinician to confidently and consistently identify
subluxations" [64]. Most chiropractic colleges offer an elective course, and
the leading proponents sponsor weekend seminars throughout the United
States. The National Board of Chiropractic Examiners 1991 job analysis
survey found that 51.2 percent of the responding chiropractors said they
used AM [38].

The claims made by AM's leaders are not modest. The Activator Methods Web site states:

> Need a program for total health?
> You may think that chiropractic care is only for back and neck pain. The truth is, chiropractic care addresses a wide variety of common health problems stemming from dysfunction in your spinal joints.
> Everyday wear and tear, old injuries, and even stress can cause your vertebrae to lose their proper position. Spinal misalignments may be a source of irritation to your nervous system, causing pain and nerve interference throughout your body.
>
> * * * * *
>
> By removing nerve interference with gentle adjustments, chiropractic allows you to enjoy optimal health without using drugs or surgery!
>
> * * * * *
>
> By coming to our office for regular chiropractic care, you'll help your body stay healthy for years to come. Regular spinal adjustments can become your body's line of defense against illness, disease, and pain. To maintain your progress and prevent re-injury, it's important that you continue your program of care.

The AM system is based on a concept of "pelvic deficiency (P.D.)"—also called "functional short leg"—which proponents define as an "apparent" difference in length, not an anatomical difference. To determine where the alleged problem is located, the practitioner holds the patient's feet in various prescribed ways while the patient lies facedown on an examining

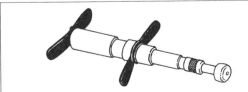

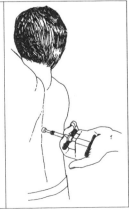

The Activator Adjusting Instrument is the most popular adjusting device used by chiropractors who believe that slight vertebral misalignments are harmful to health. It is FDA-approved as an adjusting instrument. Its patent application states the device is "'tunable' to the natural frequency of a human spine." The tip of the mallet resembles a cue tip.

This motorized adjusting instrument was designed primarily for adjusting the cervical vertebrae and works in a manner similar to the Activator mallet. One variety, called an Arthrostim, delivers high-velocity short-stroke thrusts at the rate of twelve times per second and is claimed to release trigger points and muscle spasm associated with vertebral subluxations.

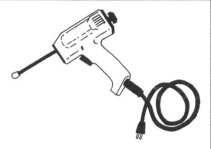

table. Other parts of the body may be tested in various other ways. If any inequality or "imbalance" is found, the practitioner taps various points along the spine, pelvis, and/or elsewhere with a handheld, spring-loaded mallet until the legs appear to be equal in length. This approach is not a method of spinal manipulation. Slight variations of hip position or normal spinal muscle tension are probably responsible for the "imbalances." Despite this, the Activator Adjusting Instrument is FDA-approved for "chiropractic adjustment of the spine and extremities."

Activator Methods thus piles one dubious concept upon another. Its leg-length tests have not been demonstrated to be reliable or to yield significant data. Nor is there any reason to believe that "pelvic deficiency" or its associated "subluxations" are pathologic conditions. Despite this, many AM practitioners tell their patients that use of an Activator mallet is a "state of the art" procedure that replaces the "old" method of manual spinal manipulation. Nothing could be further from the truth. Properly performed spinal manipulation, whether done by a physiatrist, an orthopedist, an osteopath, or a chiropractor, is always done manually. Only chiropractors use an Activator mallet. When I was in practice, I had a big problem with patients who had been convinced that their spine had tiny misalignments that required frequent correction with the tap of a mallet. Chiropractors who scare patients into believing that slight vertebral or pelvic misalignments are harmful to health are rendering a great disservice to their patients.

Contour Analysis

Moire contourography (commonly referred to as contour analysis) is a photographic technique that highlights body contours. The apparatus passes an angled light through a grid to produce a picture resembling a topographic map on the surface of the patient's body. Chiropractors who use

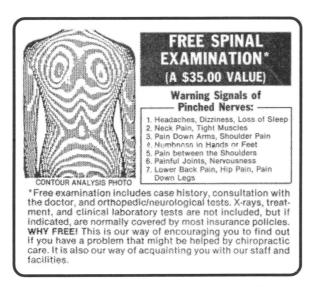

FREE SPINAL
EXAMINATION*
(A $35.00 VALUE)

Warning Signals of
Pinched Nerves:

1. Headaches, Dizziness, Loss of Sleep
2. Neck Pain, Tight Muscles
3. Pain Down Arms, Shoulder Pain
4. Numbness in Hands or Feet
5. Pain between the Shoulders
6. Painful Joints, Nervousness
7. Lower Back Pain, Hip Pain, Pain
   Down Legs

CONTOUR ANALYSIS PHOTO

*Free examination includes case history, consultation with
the doctor, and orthopedic/neurological tests. X-rays, treatment, and clinical laboratory tests are not included, but if
indicated, are normally covered by most insurance policies.
WHY FREE! This is our way of encouraging you to find out
if you have a problem that might be helped by chiropractic
care. It is also our way of acquainting you with our staff and
facilities.

Free examinations usually lead to a recommendations for extensive and
unnecessary treatment. Most of the above "warning signals" are either not
caused by pinched nerves or not appropriate for chiropractic care. Contour
analysis provides no information about pinched nerves.

contourography claim that it can detect vertebral misalignments and measure the progress of their treatment, and some offer it free as a screening test.
Careful positioning of the patient can yield results that are reproducible.
However, no scientific study has shown the test to be useful clinically [76].
Routine use should be regarded as a marketing gimmick. It is safe to assume
that everyone who undergoes "free screening" will be advised to have
treatment.

Handheld Heat Detectors

Some chiropractors claim they can detect subluxations by noticing slight
temperature differences between the sides of the spine. This idea is
traceable to chiropractic's founder, D.D. Palmer, who used the back of his
hand for this purpose. During the 1920s, Palmer's son B.J. began marketing
a handheld heat detector called the neurocalometer (see Chapter 2). Similar
devices are still used. They contain heat-detecting probes (thermocouples)
that connect to a needle gauge that registers whether points on either side
of the spine have different temperatures. Some devices are connected to a
strip-chart machine that graphs the data. To examine the patient, the

chiropractor moves the device along the spine and looks for side-to-side movement of the needle. The distributor of a modern version called the Nervo-Scope describes it as "an automatic practice builder" that will quickly pay for itself.

During the late 1950s, researchers from the Stanford Research Institute tested a neurocalometer and found that its readings were greatly influenced by how hard the instrument was pressed against the patient's skin [182]. In the 1970s, Dr. Edmund Crelin tested a ThermoScribe II and found that the handheld unit could not discriminate between heat and pressure. A colleague who tested the device on three patients with severe spine and spinal nerve disorders found that each time the test was repeated it yielded different results [52].

In 1993, a Canadian chiropractic consensus conference concluded that paraspinal measurement with thermocouple devices "has not been shown to have good discriminability, and both their validity and reliability of measurement are highly doubtful" [76]. In other words, they are worthless devices used to search for nonexistent problems.

Thermography

Thermographic devices portray small temperature differences between sides of the body as images. One type of device converts the radiated heat (infrared energy) into electronic signals that are amplified and transmitted to a monitor and/or videotape. The images may be in color or in black and white, and may be accompanied by displays of various calculations. Liquid crystal display devices exist but are not as popular. Some devices produce a printout that can be shown to the patient. An infrared thermographic examination typically costs hundreds of dollars.

Chiropractors who use thermography typically claim that it can detect nerve impingements or "nerve irritation" and is useful for monitoring the effect of chiropractic adjustments on subluxations [184]. A recent ad suggested that thermography provides "a picture of pain" and "helps the doctor and patient find and describe 'the reason for pain.'" One manufacturer has stated that thermography "attracts patients who do not wish to be x-rayed." Another has stated that it provides "comprehensive and substantive proof that each chiropractic adjustment provided some correction of a patient's problem."

The scientific view is that thermography is, at best, a research tool that would not yield useful information for day-to-day chiropractic practice. In

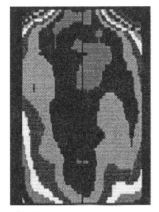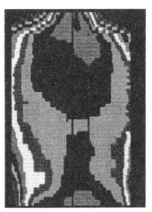

Before-and-after thermograms of the patient's body. The left-hand image purportedly shows increased heat in the left cervical area. The right-hand (post-treatment) shows "improved symmetry" in that area.

1989, the American Academy of Neurology (AAN) issued a position paper stating that thermography had not been proven useful as a screening test for patients with back or neck pain and that better tests are available for most other purpose [7]. 1994, after reviewing additional studies, an Agency for Health Care Policy and Research panel concluded:

> The one study meeting review criteria found that thermography did not accurately predict either the presence or absence of lumbar nerve root compression found at surgery. In addition, several studies have shown thermography of the lower limbs as abnormal in a substantial proportion of [symptom-free] subjects with back problems. Based on the available research evidence, thermography does not appear effective for diagnosing low back problems. [27:65]

Despite all this, colorful thermographic images are often used as a tool for selling spinal adjustments. Some chiropractors offer free thermography as a screening device. You should assume that any chiropractor who does this will find something that needs treatment.

Superfluous Testing

Many chiropractors, particularly those who emphasize treatment of personal injuries, use device-based tests to document patient progress. These include surface electromyography (SEMG), inclinometry, ultrasonography, computerized muscle-testing, and nerve-conduction studies.

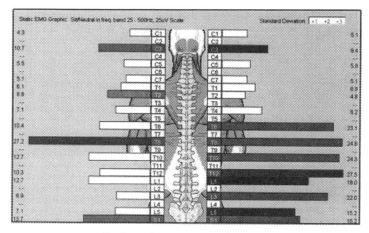

Surface electromyography report

In SEMG, the electrical activity of individual muscles or muscle groups is detected, amplified, and analyzed by a computer. The most basic information obtainable from an EMG signal is whether the tested muscle was used during a period of exertion. The test has legitimate use for analyzing certain types of performance in the workplace. However, some chiropractors claim that the test provides "an objective measurement of overall spinal health by detecting electrical activity in the muscles along the spine," enabling them to screen patients initially and to follow the progress of their treatment [104]. Some devices enable the chiropractor to interpret the results while the patient observes various markings on a schematic representation of the body on a computer screen. One such device was endorsed by a prominent chiropractor who said it was "marvelous for demonstrating the vertebral subluxation complex to the patient" and that "it helps the patients realize that when their symptoms are gone, there is still correction to be made" [69].

Ultrasonography (ultrasound testing) is performed with a device that transmits sound waves through body tissues, records the echoes as the sounds encounter body structures, and transforms the recordings into a photographic image. Diagnostic ultrasound has many useful applications in medical practice. However, some chiropractors claim that it is useful for diagnosing spine-related muscle spasm or inflammation and for following the progress of patients treated for back pain. This position is scientifically insupportable. In 1995, the American College of Radiology concluded that diagnostic ultrasound had "no proven clinical utility as a screening, diagnostic or adjunctive imaging tool" for evaluating pain, fluid in the tissues, nerve disorders or other subtle abnormalities adjacent to the spine [10]. Even the American Chiropractic Association has stated that "the application of diagnostic ultrasound in the adult spine in areas such as disk herniation, spinal stenosis and nerve root pathology is inadequately studied" and should not be done routinely [1]. Some chiropractors routinely test several segments of the spine, charging separately for each one, so that the total exceeds $1,000 on a single day.

Inclinometry provides a formal way to measure the extent to which someone can bend at the waist or flex other joints. Simply observing the patient or using a goniometer (special ruler) or an inclinometer with a gauge can provide all the information that a chiropractor would need. Computerized inclinometry, for which chiropractors typically charge hundreds of dollars, adds nothing of practical value. Similarly, computerized muscle-testing and nerve-conduction studies have legitimate medical uses, but have no practical value for chiropractic case management. The Insight 7000 Subluxation Station™ produces and graphs two types of SEMG reports plus thermal measurements and computerized inclinometry.

Some chiropractors send their x-rays for analysis by a computer that digitizes the image and computes various chiropractic angles and lines. The reports, which are expensive, rarely provide information that a skilled chiropractor cannot obtain by simply looking at the x-ray film.

To be justifiable, a diagnostic test must provide significant information that might affect patient management. In chiropractic hands, the above-mentioned high-tech tests fail to do so, and their use should be regarded as a money-making scheme. The progress of chiropractic patients can be evaluated without expensive gadgetry.

"New" Procedures

To enhance their image, chiropractors sometimes claim to have a "new" device that may not be available elsewhere. In many cases, the procedure is worthless or its value exaggerated. In 1987, for example, the Allentown (Pa.) *Morning Call* featured a local chiropractor using a Toftness Radiation Detector—three years after the FDA ordered these devices recalled. In another instance, a Florida chiropractor received television coverage when he claimed that an Electro-Acuscope would heal diseased tissue by "restoring its electromagnetic balance." When I inquired, an FDA official said that it was merely a transcutaneous electrical nerve stimulator (TENS) that was approved for treating pain but not any disease.

Recently, a television news program featured a chiropractor demonstrating "motion x-ray imaging," which was described as "the future of medicine." This procedure (cineroentgenography) produces motion pictures of spinal joints and can be used to determine the extent of joint dysfunction caused by adhesions or torn ligaments. However, it is not new and is certainly not appropriate for routine chiropractic care. Neither is videofluoroscopy, a similar procedure in which images are recorded on videotape rather than film.

You should be wary of any "new" device or procedure promoted in a chiropractic advertisement or news report.

11

A Surfeit of Techniques

Chiropractors who base their practice on correcting vertebral subluxations may employ one or more of a great variety of nonsensical techniques, some of which are performed with instruments and some of which are even applied to areas of the body unrelated to the source of a patient's symptoms. As many as 200 such techniques have been developed. *Chiropractic: An Illustrated History* lists ninety-seven of them—from Access Seminars to Zindler Reflex Technique—used in recent years [142:260]. Subluxation-based chiropractors usually feel that whatever methods they use are the most effective for restoring and maintaining health. Some even believe their work is applicable to animals.

This chapter describes a variety of approaches. Appendix D includes several more. Although most are subluxation-related, any could be of value if used to mobilize a tight spinal segment.

From Top to Bottom

The elusive "subluxation" has fostered many bizarre and antithetical diagnostic and treatment methods, some of which can be completely understood only by their entrepreneurial advocates. Some techniques are focused on the head, some on the neck, some on the lower spine, some on several spinal areas, and some on the entire spine. Yet all are claimed to "work," and some chiropractic educators suggest that all adjustive techniques that "remove nerve interference" have value. The claim that diametrically

131

opposite techniques are equally effective in improving health is absurd and suggests that few have any real value.

• "Cranial therapy" advocates claim that a rhythm exists in the flow of the fluid that surrounds the brain and spinal cord and that health problems can be diagnosed by detecting aberrations in this rhythm and corrected by manipulating the skull. Proponents claim that (a) the skull and pelvic bones move rhythmically when the person breathes; (b) the practitioner's hands can detect movement; (c) breathing influences the tension of the membranes (dura) that surround the brain and spinal cord; and (d) all other body systems are directly and indirectly related to this respiratory system. However, cerebrospinal fluid has no palpable rhythm and cranial bones cannot be manipulated because they fuse during infancy.

Cranial techniques can be used alone or as part of a system called Sacro-occipital Technique (SOT), which holds that rhythmic motion of the sacral bones is also important. Its founder believed that each vertebra is related to a visceral area, thus affecting all the internal organs [54]. SOT practitioners check leg lengths to look for "lumbar instability" and subluxation patterns and use padded lumbar wedges and full-spine adjusting techniques to "balance the pelvis."

• Palmer Upper Cervical Technique was introduced by B.J. Palmer in the 1930s but is still practiced today. The practitioner measures supposed atlas-axis misalignments and uses a toggle recoil technique in which a quick thrust is applied to the side of the neck and then is quickly withdrawn. Correcting the alignment of the atlas or the axis at the top of the spine will supposedly correct subluxations and other problems from the neck down. In 1958, Palmer maintained that the only place a primary causative vertebral subluxation can occur is in the atlas area, and that atlas realignment was necessary before other (secondary) subluxations could be corrected. Many varieties of upper cervical approaches exist. In addition to manual manipulation, in which the heel of the hand is applied to the side of the neck, they may use a handheld device or tabletop stylus machine to adjust the atlas.

• Advocates of Neural Organization Technique (N.O.T.) claim that learning disorders, childhood psychoses, mental retardation, attention deficit disorder, cerebral palsy, bedwetting, colorblindness, scoliosis, epilepsy, and several other conditions are related to muscle imbalances caused by misaligned skull bones. Its developer, Carl Ferreri, D.C., states that the technique is based on applied kinesiology, sacro-occipital technique, cranial technique, sacro-cranial technique, chiropractic, acupuncture, and his own observations. It includes leg-length testing (for "atlas subluxations"),

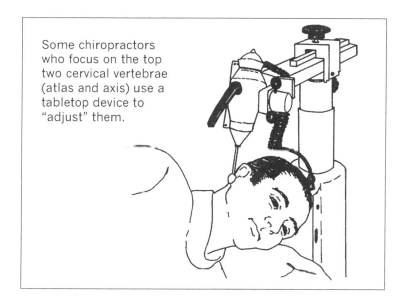

Some chiropractors who focus on the top two cervical vertebrae (atlas and axis) use a tabletop device to "adjust" them.

muscle-testing, checking how the tongue moves when protruded, and so many nonstandard "reflex" tests that it is difficult to summarize. N.O.T.'s advocates claim to correct "blocked neural pathways" by "adjusting" the bones of the skull with pressure to various parts of the head. The vice-president of one N.O.T. organization claims that "Cranial or head injury is probably the single most undiagnosed, and therefore untreated physical problem on the face of the earth" [158].

In the late 1980s, N.O.T. was severely criticized after the Del Norte (California) Unified School District sponsored a "research project" to test N.O.T.'s effect on children with epilepsy, Down syndrome, cerebral palsy, dyslexia, and various other learning disorders. A 1988 report in *Hippocrates* magazine described how many children were forced to endure pain when chiropractors pressed against their skull, roof of the mouth, and eyes. One parent complained that pressure against her son's eye sockets had caused a seizure [47]. In 1991, a jury ordered Ferreri to pay $565,000 in damages to seven children and their parents who had filed suit for physical and emotional pain related to the treatment. Two others settled out of court for a total of $207,000.

• In the Gonstead Method, the pelvis and sacrum are analyzed to help locate primary and secondary subluxations in the spine. Subluxations are then confirmed by x-ray examination, skin temperature readings, and motion palpation. Correction of the primary subluxation is supposed to result in automatic correction of secondary subluxations. According to this theory, repeated adjustment of the secondary subluxations can be avoided by first correcting the primary subluxations. This treatment method is used more to restore and maintain health than to treat back pain.

• Logan Basic Technique is based on the belief that subluxations anywhere in the spine occur as a result of body distortions caused by leg-length inequality, sacral subluxation, or by wedging of the fifth lumbar vertebra. The patient is analyzed for subluxations by examining the sacrum and leg length in the standing position and by x-ray examination. Before spinal corrections are made, the sacrum is "adjusted" by placing thumb pressure on the sacrotuberous ligament or on the apex of the sacrum, probing a buttock on one side. The technique's founder maintained that "it is absolutely necessary to restore the sacrum to normal position and relationship with articulating bones to effectively reduce curvatures, sub-luxations, and disease" [117].

• The meric system relates diseases and body organs to subluxations at specific levels of the spine. Chiropractors who follow this system usually display charts showing which organs or conditions are supposedly related to which spinal segments. Patients treated with the meric system will often get adjustments at their "kidney place," "stomach place," or some other specific spot, depending upon what kind of trouble they are having.

• Directional Nonforce Technique (DNFT) is a method of diagnosing and correcting subluxations by applying thumb pressure to the spine in certain directions and checking leg length, which supposedly changes when correction is made. Disk corrections are made by lightly thrusting between the vertebrae with a $3/8$-inch wood dowel. Subluxations are located without the use of x-ray examination, and correction is made without popping the vertebrae. Although advocates claim that a subluxation can often be corrected with one treatment with a light thumb thrust, they recommend preventive-maintenance adjustments every one to four months. This technique is ideal for chiropractors who want to treat symptom-free patients on a regular basis with a harmless —though useless—method.

• Thompson Terminal Point Technique requires a special table with sections that drop a short distance when a thrust or adjustment is applied to the spine. The sudden release of the supporting cushion is supposed to use kinetic energy to facilitate the adjustment and make it easier for the chiropractor. To determine whether back-related subluxations are present, leg length is compared in supine and prone positions, with the legs straight and with the knees bent. Cervical subluxations are located by comparing leg length while the head is turned to one side or the other.

• Diversified Technique uses a variety of adjustive techniques to detect subluxations and to create motion in a vertebral joint. Some of these mobilizing techniques are effective in the treatment of back pain. Chiropractors who use diversified technique are more likely to offer appropriate hands-on spinal manipulation than those who use a "special technique."

• Cox Flexion-Distraction Technique is a mechanically assisted manipulative technique in which a special table is used to enhance manual traction applied to specific spinal segments. The patient is placed facedown on the table, with both ankles secured at the foot of the table. The forward part of the table is then lowered to produce a flexion-type traction. Manual pressure is applied to the spine to produce localized traction or distraction in a specific joint or disk. This approach, developed in recent years as a method of treating back pain, makes sense when its use is appropriate and indicated. But it should not be used when it seems to aggravate back pain. Patients who have acute back pain and who have difficulty getting out of bed and who may have swelling in a joint may be unable to get off the table and walk after a painful joint has been repeatedly stretched. Although the technique's developer described its purposes in standard physiologic terms, some chiropractors use it to treat "subluxations."

The 4,385 full-time chiropractors who responded to the 1991 National Board of Chiropractic Examiners survey said that they used an average of 5.7 techniques. The reported percentages for individual techniques included: diversified, 91.1 percent; Gonstead, 54.8 percent; Cox, 52.7 percent; Thompson, 43 percent; SOT, 41.3 percent; Logan Basic, 30 percent; cranial therapy, 27.2 percent; Palmer upper cervical, 26 percent; and meric, 23.4 percent [38].

Animal Chiropractic

Although chiropractic education does not deal with animals, and veterinary schools do not teach manipulation, some members of both professions claim that spinal adjustments can benefit animals as well as humans. The American Veterinary Chiropractic Association (AVCA) of Port Byron, Illinois, which has members from both professions, offers courses ranging from a one-day seminar in animal adjusting to a 150-hour course leading to "certification" in animal chiropractic.

The rhetoric of "animal chiropractic" advocates resembles that of subluxation-based chiropractors. AVCA founder Sharon Willoughby, D.V.M., D.C., states, for example:

> For the veterinarian who understands the elements of holistic
> practice and the philosophy of chiropractic, every patient becomes
> a possible chiropractic patient. Every examination should include
> a spinal examination, and every treatment protocol should include
> an adjustment if necessary. [201]

"Holistic veterinarian" Joyce C. Harmon, D.V.M., asserts:

> Many practitioners believe that the spine is not worth checking
> unless a musculoskeletal problem is being examined; however,
> every cell in the body has a nerve supply originating in the nervous
> system. The nervous system is therefore important to the health of
> all organ systems, and a chiropractic examination is advised for
> every patient. . . .
> Chiropractic is an excellent way to build a veterinary practice
> because it includes preventive care after the initial problem is
> solved. [73]

One Wisconsin chiropractor asserts that "Chiropractic care offers a
natural, drug-free adjunct to . . . total health care" and is suitable for treating
cats, dogs, and horses for: back, neck, leg, or tail pain; carpal tunnel
syndrome; degenerative arthritis; disk problems; head tilt; injuries resulting
from slips and falls; TMJ problems; difficulty chewing; sudden changes in
behavior or personality; uneven muscle development; uneven pelvis or
hips; weight loss due to pain; "a look of apprehension or pain in the facial
expression"; and various other problems [99].

David V. Ramey, D.V.M., co-chairman of Quackwatch's Task Force
on Animal Quackery, has responded to the above claims:

> The forces on the spine of an animal that walks on four limbs are
> quite different from those of one that walks on two. Thus, even if
> human chiropractic theories were plausible, direct application to
> animals might not be warranted. For example, since the vertebrae
> of horses are the size of the adult fist and surrounded by muscle,
> tendon, and ligament layers several inches thick, it seems reason-
> able to wonder whether vertebrae can actually be manipulated.
> Of course, all of these concerns beg the question of whether
> "adjusting" dogs, cats, or horses really works. No scientific studies
> show that chiropractic adjustment does anything useful in any
> animal. It may be reasonable to surmise that moving an animal's
> limbs around, massaging its muscles, or giving it any sort of
> attention might be well-received by the animal, but there is no
> evidence that such attention can improve health. Furthermore, no
> published study has ever shown how a chiropractic-related prob-
> lem can be diagnosed in animals or how treatment success can be
> determined.

There are also potential dangers. Chiropractic manipulation in humans usually entails short, thrusting movements applied at segments of the spine or at specific joints. Horses have been injured by overly aggressive maneuvers described as animal "chiropractic." Manipulating the spine of a dog with a degenerative disk carries the risk of severe and permanent harm to the spinal cord. . . . Dramatic movements that stretch beyond the limits of normal range of motion — for example, the lifting of a horse's hind leg over its back—are potentially harmful. . . .

From a legal perspective, practicing on animals is restricted to veterinarians in all states. Technically, chiropractors may work on animals under the direct supervision of a veterinarian if the veterinarian feels that such treatment is warranted. However, in doing so, the chiropractor is working as an unlicensed veterinary technician. . . . Accordingly, anyone manipulating animals who is not a veterinarian or working under direct veterinary supervision is likely to be breaking current laws.

The Bottom Line

Effective spinal manipulation is usually performed by hand over the area of the pain. But spinal manipulation is only one of several methods of treating back or neck problems. In some cases, rest or exercise may be all that is needed. In others, especially those involving simple muscle strain, physical therapy, such as ultrasound or electrical stimulation, may be more effective. When a spinal joint loses mobility, hands-on spinal manipulation may be the treatment of choice. Chiropractors whose treatment armamentarium includes physical therapy as well as manipulation will be better able to select an appropriate treatment method than subluxation-based "straight chiropractors" who offer only spinal adjustments.

The hands-on manipulation used by chiropractors is similar to that used by osteopaths, physical therapists, and other science-based professionals. Chiropractors who "adjust" only the atlas or sacrum, who use an instrument to correct "subluxations," or who base their treatment on such diagnostic gadgetry as thermography or surface electromyography, are more likely to miss the mark. Those who use a variety of such techniques are simply offering a greater amount of nonsense. None of them are as scientifically grounded as a practitioner—chiropractic or medical—who uses simple hands-on manipulation for relieving back pain or for restoring mobility to specific spinal segments.

12

Homeopathy, Chinese Medicine, and Herbs

"Alternative health care," though currently quite popular, is a haven for unproven and implausible healing methods based on metaphysical belief systems. Many chiropractors embrace such beliefs, and most states permit chiropractors to use various "alternative" methods [114].

This chapter discusses homeopathy and traditional Chinese medicine (TCM), both of which resemble subluxation-based chiropractic in at least one way. True believers in all three assert that bodily functions depend on a "life force" that the scientific community does not acknowledge. Subluxation-based chiropractors claim to assist the body's "Innate Intelligence" by adjusting the patient's spine. Homeopaths postulate that illness is due to a disturbance of the body's "vital force," which they can correct with highly diluted remedies. TCM practitioners attribute disease to imbalance in the flow of "life energy" (*Qi*), which they can "balance" with acupuncture or herbs. Herbs, of course, can also be prescribed for their pharmacologic actions, but whether chiropractors should be involved with them is another matter.

Chiropractors and Homeopathy

Homeopathy was devised by a German physician named Samuel Hahnemann. In 1796, he noticed during experiments on himself that, after taking cinchona bark (the source of the malaria remedy quinine), he experienced symptoms similar to those of patients with malaria. Like

139

D.D. Palmer, he soon drew a sweeping conclusion that became the core principle of a new healing system. After further tests on himself, his family, and his friends, Hahnemann concluded that substances that cause symptoms in healthy people are effective against conditions that have those symptoms. He also noted that repeatedly diluting and shaking seemed to make his remedies more potent.

Homeopathic products are derived from minerals, plants, and various other "natural" substances. Soluble sources are diluted with distilled water and/or alcohol. Insoluble sources are pulverized and mixed with milk sugar. One part of the diluted mixture is diluted again, and the process is repeated to reach the desired concentration. The basis for formulating these products is not clinical testing but homeopathic "provings," during which substances are administered to healthy people who record their thoughts and physical sensations over various periods of time. Most provings have not followed standard protocols, and many were done more than a century ago when there was little understanding of the placebo effect or the natural variability of symptoms over time [168]. Nevertheless, the results were compiled into reference books called *materia medica,* which contain long lists of symptoms claimed to be associated with each substance. Proponents also claim that even if the dilution is so great that no molecule of original substance remains, an "essence" of the active ingredient persists and can stimulate the body's recuperative powers.

Homeopathy remedies are selected in several ways. "Classical" homeopaths tailor their prescriptions to the individual patient, based on a detailed history that includes questions about how the patient reacts to the weather and other environmental characteristics. However, most practitioners prescribe products targeted at the patient's symptoms or disease, and some select remedies with the help of a galvanometer purported to measure "electromagnetic energy imbalances."

A 1991 survey by the National Board of Chiropractic Examiners found that 36.9 percent of those who responded said that they had prescribed homeopathic remedies within the previous two years. Although no systematic study has been published, most of them probably use a "cookbook" approach in which they match the remedies as indicated in a manual distributed by a manufacturer.

The leading chiropractic supplier appears to be King Bio Pharmaceuticals, of Ashville, North Carolina. Its president, Frank J. King, N.D., D.C., writes regularly in chiropractic trade publications and maintains a Web site. In an interview titled "The Marriage of Chiropractic and Homeopathy," he stated:

Homeopathy does not treat diseases per se. Homeopathy activates the body's own healing processes in both the physical and mental/emotional levels. The range of problems in which homeopathy can be effectively utilized is extensive and includes first aid, illnesses, and all manner of chronic conditions. We have found homeopathy to be most effective in correcting . . . anorexia and bulimia, breast cysts, infertility, menopause, feminine discharge, PMS, male disorders, bedwetting, colic, earaches, learning disabilities, hyperactivity, parasites, swollen tonsils, teething, digestive disorders, gout, arthritis, migraines, sinus, immune disorders, acne, asthma, bladder incontinence, colds and flu, fatigue syndromes, herpes, hypoglycemia, kidney and bladder complaints, lung disorders, memory, motion sickness, chronic skin disorders, laryngitis, warts, weight control, anxiety, depression, and insomnia. [105]

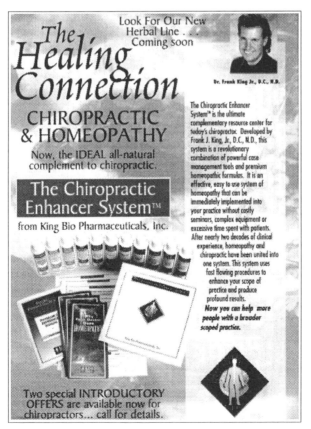

Frank King, Jr., D.C., N.D., states that "homeopathy and chiropractic have been united into one system. . . . Now you can help people with a broader scoped practice."

King states that the appropriate remedy "can provide fast, gentle relief, often within minutes or even seconds in certain cases" and that "many successful chiropractors who use homeopathy see over 200 patients per day on a long term basis" [106]. His Web site features a patient self-appraisal form that suggests a product for each of about fifty problems. His online professional repertory suggests products for angina, cataracts, epilepsy, "insanity," suicidal tendencies, tumors, and more than 250 other conditions, most of which are very far outside the scope of rational chiropractic practice.

In order for homeopathy to work as its proponents claim, all of the following would have to be true:

- Substances that cause symptoms in healthy people can cure these symptoms in sick people.
- The smaller the amount, the more potent the remedy.
- Substances can cure people even if completely absent.
- The usefulness of the original substances can be determined by having people take nonstandardized amounts and record their symptoms over nonstandard periods of time.

None of the above makes any sense, and no homeopathic remedy has even been proven to cure anything [56,95]. In fact, the vast majority of products marketed today have never been clinically tested. Although a quirk in federal law permits homeopathic products to be sold, neither the scientific community nor the FDA recognizes them as effective. Curiously, National College of Chiropractic, which is one of chiropractic's relatively science-based schools, offers a "diplomate" program in homeopathy through its postgraduate division.

Chiropractic's "Perfect Partner"?

Traditional Chinese medicine (TCM) is an elaborate system of folk practices rooted in mysticism. Its practitioners claim that the body's "vital energy" (*Qi* or *chi*) circulates through hypothetical channels ("meridians") that branch to bodily organs and functions. They also claim that ill health is caused by "imbalance" of *Qi*, and that acupuncture restores health by stimulating and rebalancing its flow. This is done by inserting needles at "acupuncture points" located throughout the body. A low-frequency current may be applied to the needles to produce greater stimulation. TCM practitioners typically prescribe many herbs. As noted in a booklet from Integrated Medicine Communications:

To determine what is causing illness, a TCM practitioner looks for imbalances in heat/cold, moisture/dryness, and excess/deficiency in . . . qi, blood, and moisture. The causes of these imbalances are determined by five organ networks: the liver, heart, spleen, lungs, and kidneys. Each organ network has the capability to generate wind, heat, dampness, dryness, and cold; each corresponds to five planes: wood, fire, earth, metal, and water; and each correlates to five cycles of development, five seasons, five climates, and five personality types. When the organ networks are out of balance or are functioning in the absence of sufficient qi, illness ensues. [11]

Chiropractic interest in acupuncture is significant. The 1991 NBCE survey found that 11.8% of respondents said they practiced acupuncture [38]. If that figure is still accurate, more than 5,000 chiropractors are offering acupuncture today.

In March 1998, the *Journal of the American Chiropractic Association (JACA)* published a five-part series called "Acupuncture: Chiropractic's Perfect Partner?" An accompanying glossary described acupuncture's goal as "to return the body to health by stimulating the flow of its natural health-promoting energies." One article was provided by David Wells, D.C, L.Ac., director of oriental medicine for Landmark Health Care, a California-based company that offers "alternative" managed care. He wrote:

In my experience, acupuncture is a brilliant adjunct in the treatment of musculoskeletal injury. . . . Acupuncture also opens the door to treatment of a wide variety of organic and metabolic complaints— allergies, asthma, dysmenorrhea, PMS, gastritis, colitis, cystitis, upper respiratory infections, stroke, and addictions. [195]

Another contributor to the issue stated:

The unique skill of chiropractic is our ability to palpate, detect, and correct spinal vertebral subluxations after a consultation and examination. . . . The level of spinal subluxation for a particular health condition often matches the corresponding . . . acupuncture point." [78]

TCM diagnosis and treatment does not correspond to science-based concepts of body physiology. *Qi,* "meridians," and "acupuncture points" have never been scientifically demonstrated to exist. *Qi* is TCM's equivalent of chiropractic's "Innate Intelligence," and meridians and acupuncture points are as elusive as chiropractic's subluxations. Medical science recognizes only one pulse, corresponding to the heartbeat, which can be felt in the wrist and many other places throughout the body. TCM practitioners check six alleged pulses at each wrist and identify more than twenty-five alleged pulse qualities that supposedly reflect the type of imbalance, the condition of each organ system, and the status of the patient's *Qi*. TCM practitioners also use "tongue diagnosis" to help determine patterns of "body harmony or disharmony." As described by acupuncturist Misha Ruth Cohen, author of *The Chinese Way to Healing: Many Paths to Wholeness*:

> The Chinese medicine doctor looks at the color of the tongue body, its size and shape, the color and thickness of its coating or fur, locations of abnormalities, and moistness or dryness of the tongue body and fur. These signs reveal not only overall states of health but correlate to specific organ functions and disharmonies, especially in the digestive system. [41]

Cohen states, for example:

> A trembling, pale tongue indicates Deficient Qi. A flaccid tongue that is pale often reveals extreme Qi or Xue Deficiency. A flaccid tongue that is deep red reveals severe Yin Deficiency. A trembling, red tongue indicates interior Wind. If the tongue sits off-center in the mouth, early or full-blown Wind stroke may be present. A rigid tongue accompanies an Exterior Pernicious Influence and fever. This may indicate the invasion of the Pericardium by Heat and Mucus Obstructing the Heart Qi. [41]

A Texas chiropractor's Web site provides yet another glimpse at TCM's metaphysical mumbo-jumbo:

> As with acupuncture, herbalism works to relieve abnormalities which negatively affect the proper flow of chi along your meridians. Herbalism can be used as an adjunct to, or in some cases, a substitute for, acupuncture. While acupuncture is viewed as yang because it works from the external in, herbalism is seen as yin because it works from the internal out. Because of this dichotomous relationship, the two therapies work well in combination together. In cases where acupuncture cannot be replaced, but the patient is weak and has little chi with which acupuncture can work, herbalism can often increase the patient's energy flow. [205]

Although acupuncture may have some usefulness for pain relief, the National Council Against Health Fraud has concluded: (a) its theory and practice are based on primitive and fanciful concepts of health and disease that bear no relationship to present scientific knowledge; and (b) research has not demonstrated effectiveness against any disease [157]. The herbs associated with TCM are not regulated for safety, potency, or effectiveness. In short, patients going to TCM practitioners—whether chiropractors or not—are unlikely to be treated rationally.

"Electrodiagnostic" Testing

Some chiropractors—probably a few hundred—use "electrodiagnostic" devices to help determine what treatment to administer. The procedure, which is called "electroacupuncture of Voll" ("EAV") or electrodermal testing, is said to detect "imbalances in the flow of electro-magnetic energy" along acupuncture meridians. Sometimes the procedure is misrepresented as "stress testing." The currently used devices include Avatar System, Body Scan 2010, Computron, DiagnoMètre, Eclosion, LISTEN System, MORA, Omega AcuBase, and Vegatest. Dr. Stephen Barrett has noted:

> Actually, they are little more than fancy galvanometers that measure electrical resistance of the patient's skin when touched by a probe. One wire from the device goes to a brass cylinder covered by moist gauze, which the patient holds in one hand. A second wire is connected to a probe, which the operator touches to "acupuncture points" on the patient's other hand or a foot. This completes a low-voltage circuit and the device registers the flow of current.
>
> The information is then relayed to a gauge or computer screen that provides a numerical readout on a scale of 0 to 100. . . . The size of the number actually depends on how hard the probe is pressed against the patient's skin. [20]

The findings are then used to prescribe homeopathic remedies, acupuncture, dietary change, vitamin supplements, and/or spinal adjustments. These devices cannot be legally marketed in the United States for diagnostic or treatment purposes, but state and federal agencies have done little to curtail their use.

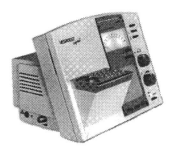 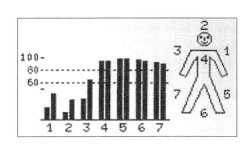

A current Vegatest model feeds data to a printer that produces graphs like the one pictured here. The accompanying report concludes that this fifty-year-old woman has "fatigue state, infection susceptibility, but with positive tendency, since regulating to norm . . . problem with the excretory organs, blockage in the thorax . . . allergic tendency and hormonal stress as well as susceptibility to head congestion."

Chiropractors and Herbal Medicine

To my knowledge, no published study has determined how many chiropractors prescribe herbs, why they prescribe them, or where they obtain the information that guides them. It is clear, however, that several dozen manufacturers are marketing herbs to chiropractors, and that some have been doing it for many years. Phytopharmica, of Green Bay, Wisconsin, for example, markets "natural" products through chiropractors and other health professionals. Its 1995 catalog includes *Adren-Plus, CircuMax, FemTone, MascuPlex, SinuClear,* and *Utero-Tone,* and more than fifty other herbal products. The products currently marketed by PhysioLogics, of Boulder, Colorado, include *Paraclear* (to help kill and expel parasites), *RejuVeinate* (for vein health), *Resphora* ("to support normal breathing"), *Thyroid Support Formula,* and *VitaCardia.* Since the law limits what manufacturers can claim directly, some sponsor seminars or publications that disseminate the claims for them.

Stripped of their metaphysical trappings, herbs are drugs. To make a rational decision about any drug, it is necessary to know what it contains, whether it is safe, and whether it has been demonstrated to be as good or better than other drugs available for the same purpose. For most herbal products this information is incomplete or unavailable [21]. The fact that large pharmaceutical companies have begun marketing a few herbs will probably lead to increased research and improved product standardization. However, chiropractors are not trained to diagnose or treat the broad spectrum of disease, and most know very little about the pharmacology of drugs, whether standard or herbal. For these reasons, I do not believe that chiropractors should prescribe herbs.

Misplaced Priorities

Despite accumulating scientific support for the use of spinal manipulation for treating back and neck pain, many chiropractors continue to dabble in metaphysical methods that parallel subluxation theory. Chiropractors should, of course, stick with what they do best—the use of manipulation and other physical treatment methods for musculoskeletal problems. But until the current craze for "alternative" methods has run its course, it seems likely that the chiropractic profession will be more influenced by the kindred spirits of "alternative medicine" than by the iconoclastic laws of the physical sciences.

13

What a Rational Chiropractor
Can Do for You

Spinal manipulation can relieve some types of back and neck pain and other conditions related to tightness and loss of mobility, such as tension headache or aching in muscles and joints. We also know that massage may be as effective as cervical manipulation in relieving tension headache. And physical therapy may be as effective as spinal manipulation in long-term relief of back pain. Rational chiropractors can offer all of these modalities, when appropriate, and thus provide patients with a choice. They may also offer basic advice about nutrition, weight loss, exercise, ergonomics, relaxation techniques, body mechanics, home care (such as use of hot or cold packs), massage, and other self-help measures that might help relieve or prevent aches and pains.

Science-based chiropractors make appropriate judgments about the nature of their patients' problems, determine whether these problems lie within their scope, and make appropriate referrals for problems that do not. If you can find one who uses manipulation and physical therapy appropriately and who is willing to coordinate with your personal physician, you can benefit from the best that both have to offer. Here are some examples of patients who benefited from chiropractic care:

- John C, age thirty-three, had never had back pain. One day, however, his lower back began to hurt after he spent several hours working under the hood of his car. When he stood or walked around, his low-back muscles hurt and felt stiff and tight. He was comfortable when lying down or sitting. John had no history of disease or previous injury. The diagnosis was simple lumbar strain. No x-ray examination was needed. I advised him to rest at home and to apply hot packs after two days. His symptoms subsided after four days, and he needed no further treatment.

• Lewis D, a twenty-four-year-old construction worker, hurt his back lifting heavy lumber. Three days later, he visited my office complaining of acute low-back pain and muscle spasm that made it difficult for him to get up and down. Since he had had several previous episodes, I x-rayed his spine and found that his fifth lumbar vertebra was positioned slightly more forward than the sacral bone below it, a congenital condition called spondylolisthesis. The diagnosis was lumbosacral strain complicated by this joint abnormality. After a few days of rest and treatment with cold packs at home, Lewis returned for manipulation and physical therapy two or three times a week. After three weeks, his symptoms had eased enough to permit him to return to work on light duty. In three more weeks, he was well enough to be released from care.

• Susan C, a thirty-year-old hairdresser, had chronic neck and upper back pain. Often, after long hours at work, the muscles in her neck and upper back ached and were sore and sensitive, especially between her shoulder blades. She had been experiencing these symptoms for years and had no significant history of injury or illness. Medical examination was always negative. Susan's diagnosis was posture-related myofascitis (inflammation of muscles and their fascial covering). When her symptoms were worse than usual, she would come in a couple of times a week for manipulation and physical therapy, which usually consisted of ultrasound and electrical stimulation or massage, for symptomatic relief. I instructed her in the use of exercises designed to strengthen the supporting muscles in her neck and upper back. Because of chronic inflammation caused by postural imbalance and work strain, Susan elected to return for treatment when she felt she needed it.

• Albert T, a fifty-four-year-old retired stockbroker, leaned over one day and felt a "catch" in his lower back. He could not straighten up completely and was tilted slightly to one side. He could rotate his spine to the left but not to the right. He had no significant history of disease or injury. A gentle side-posture manipulation, with Albert lying on his left side, unlocked a binding spinal joint and provided immediate relief of symptoms with restoration of normal movement. No further treatment was needed. The fact that a single manipulation sometimes provides dramatic relief has helped to boost chiropractic's reputation.

• Martha D, age seventy-five, suddenly developed pain in her upper back when she moved a heavy piece of furniture. She had a slight hump in her thoracic spine, and she felt pain when I tapped on her most prominent vertebra. Because of her age and her history of taking cortisone for arthritis, I obtained x-rays. The diagnosis was osteoporosis with crush fracture of a mid-thoracic vertebra, a condition that neither manipulation nor physical therapy could remedy. I referred her to an orthopedic specialist who prescribed medication and supplements to help strengthen her bones.

• Alice P, a fifty-year-old bookkeeper, had had surgery for uterine cancer. Four years afterward, she began to have constant back pain that was not relieved by rest. She visited my office asking for spinal adjustments. When Alice gave me her history and described her symptoms, I immediately sent her to her family physician who could initiate a search for metastatic cancer. She called back later to report that she had bone cancer and was seeing a cancer specialist.

• Frances R, a forty-eight-year-old dental assistant, reported that she was limping because of pain in her right thigh and knee, which she felt was caused by a pinched nerve. When examination of her reflexes and the structures of her right thigh and knee did not reveal any significant findings, I realized that pain was being referred down the front of her thigh from a hip-socket problem. Her physical examination revealed decreased range of motion of her right hip, and an x-ray examination showed necrosis (crumbling) of the top of the leg bone inside the hip joint. I referred her to an orthopedic surgeon who determined that she would eventually need hip-replacement surgery.

• Jack D., a thirty-year-old electrician, attempted to slide a 300-pound roll of wire off the bed of a truck. During the exertion, he felt severe pain in his lower back and in both legs and fell to the ground, totally incapacitated. Several days later, he came to my office complaining of back pain along with pain and weakness in both legs. The reflexes in his right leg and foot were diminished, and he could not lift the front of his foot, resulting in a "foot drop" that caused his foot to flop when he walked. I immediately referred him to a neurosurgeon who found spinal canal encroachment caused by two severely herniated lower lumbar disks near the nerves supplying his bladder and anal sphincters. Both disk protrusions were surgically removed. Spinal manipulation in this case could have had disastrous results, possibly causing permanent loss of bladder and bowel control.

Diagnosis Essential

Many more examples of back-pain management could be given, covering a great variety of conditions in persons of all ages. But the above are sufficient to demonstrate that, while some types of back pain can benefit from spinal manipulation, not every patient who sees a chiropractor needs it. And they illustrate why proper diagnosis should precede treatment of any type. This is why, if you consult a chiropractor, it is crucial to choose one who can make an appropriate diagnosis, uses spinal manipulation only when indicated, does not order unnecessary x-rays, and refers to an appropriate physician when needed. Chiropractors whose practice is not based on subluxation theory are in the best position to judge whether your problem requires medical treatment. Never rely upon the diagnosis of a straight chiropractor or one who "specializes" in such fields as internal medicine, neurology, or pediatrics.

Back-pain sufferers who have been diagnosed with musculoskeletal pain and have reservations about spinal manipulation should ask their physician whether a referral for physical therapy is appropriate for their condition. (Actually, many chiropractors offer both.) A study published in the October 8, 1998, issue of the *New England Journal of Medicine* found that the long-term effectiveness of chiropractic manipulation was no better than the McKenzie method of physical therapy (an exercise program) [35]. However, many patients have told me that manipulation was more effective in providing immediate relief.

Manipulation vs. Mobilization

Manipulation and mobilization are used primarily in the treatment of conditions related to mechanical-type problems in joints and muscles. Manipulation is a hands-on procedure used to restore normal movement by loosening joints and stretching tight muscles. In some cases, manipulation will restore normal movement by unlocking a joint or by breaking down adhesions. A popping sound often occurs when a spinal joint is stretched a little beyond its normal range of motion. Mobilization simply stretches soft tissues by moving joints through a full range of movement. Mobilization can increase the range of motion of the arms, legs, and shoulders, but manipulation may be more effective in relieving pain and restoring normal movement in the spinal joints.

Any portion of the spine that is tight, stiff, or painful on movement might benefit from appropriate manipulation. Different methods are used in different portions of the spine, since joint structure and the direction of movement in the neck and upper back differ from those of the lower back. For example: neck manipulation might be done while the patient sits on a stool; upper-back manipulation might be done while the patient lies facedown; and lower-back manipulation might be done while the patient lies on one side. Dozens of manipulative techniques can be used to meet the special needs of patients who must be positioned one way or another. Tables with specially designed cushions are used to support patients in certain postures.

Neck Manipulation

Manipulation may improve the mobility of a cervical spine that has been stiffened by osteoarthritis or by scar tissue from an old injury. Disk degeneration caused by wear and tear or by injury is a common cause of loss of range of motion in the cervical spine and can often benefit from manipulation. Neck manipulation or mobilization may improve range of motion and provide relief for neck pain and muscle-tension headache. But remember that benefit must be weighed against risk. As noted in Chapter 7, neck manipulation should not be used unless symptoms indicate a specific need for it. It should be done gently with care to avoid excessive rotation that could damage the patient's vertebral artery. Neck manipulation should not be done immediately after an injury that causes acute neck pain. When the acute pain subsides, usually after a few days, manipulation may be useful to relieve fixations and restore normal joint mobility. Once the patient is symptom-free, it should be discontinued.

Neck manipulation is safest when neck rotation does not exceed 50 degrees. When rotation is not indicated or appropriate, special techniques can be used with the patient in a facedown position so that manipulative traction can be applied or there can be thumb contact with specific spinal segments.

Patients with pain caused by acute inflammation, as occurs in rheumatoid arthritis or spondylitis, will rarely benefit from neck manipulation. Damage to upper cervical connective tissues in rheumatoid arthritis can also be a contraindication. When in doubt about whether to undergo neck manipulation, check with an orthopedist. A competent chiropractor should not object to your seeing a specialist for a second opinion.

Tension headaches, often called muscle-contraction headaches, may benefit from manipulation that loosens joints and stretches tight neck muscles. Some chiropractic case reports suggest that migraine headache can be relieved with cervical manipulation. However, manipulation is unlikely to relieve true migraine.

Any kind of persistent headache should be brought to the attention of your family physician or a neurologist. And so should any headache accompanied by fever, vomiting, weakness, a change in speech or vision, or any other unexplained symptoms. Severe headaches may require medical attention for pain relief.

Before submitting to the risk of cervical manipulation for the treatment of headache, it is essential to determine whether the problem might be caused by a sinus infection, food sensitivity, a brain tumor, or another cause unrelated to the cervical spine. Fortunately, most headaches are of the simple tension or muscle-contraction variety. So there is a good chance that simple massage or stretching of neck muscles will relieve them.

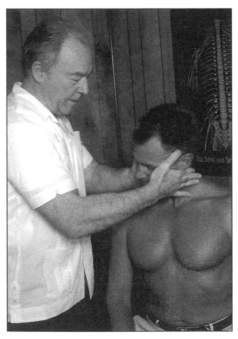

Neck manipulation should be used only when indicated and never as a preventive measure in a patient who has no symptoms.

A study published in 1998 in the *Journal of the American Medical Association* found that neck manipulation may be no more effective than massage for treating episodic or recurring tension headache [30]. Thus people with frequent tension headaches might want to try massage rather than risk injury from cervical manipulation. Here are two cases illustrating some of the above points:

• Jim D, a sixty-two-year-old accountant, had suffered from tension headaches for many years. Job stress, postural strain, and cervical arthritis were causing his neck muscles to be chronically tight, which resulted in episodes of neck pain and headache. Physical examination revealed that he was able to rotate his neck only about halfway. X-ray examination revealed moderate cervical osteoarthritis with disk degeneration. Because of previous experiences with chiropractors and osteopaths, Jim requested cervical manipulation, since he felt that such treatment was most effective in relieving his neck pain as well as his headache. The stiffness and decreased range of motion indicated that manipulation might indeed be more helpful than massage of his neck muscles. Following preliminary treatment with manual cervical traction and electrical stimulation of his neck and upper-back muscles, I gently manipulated his neck. This maneuver resulted in dramatic and immediate relief of neck pain, with a temporary increase in cervical rotation to about two-thirds normal. His tension headache then gradually subsided over a period of a few hours. When his symptoms returned, Jim would return for treatment that included cervical manipulation—sometimes once or twice a month, sometimes a few times a year.

• Shannon H, a thirty-five-year-old medical secretary, consulted me for help with pain in her neck. She had a history of infections and allergies that had affected her sinuses. The sinus infections were often accompanied by pain at the base of her skull and behind her left eye. My examination of her neck found normal movement with no apparent muscle spasm or tension. Her temperature was slightly elevated. I concluded that her neck pain was related to her sinus difficulty and referred her to an ear, nose, and throat specialist who confirmed that she had a clogged sinus and treated it accordingly.

Up and Down the Back

Pain in the upper and lower portions of the spine can often be treated successfully with manipulation and physical therapy. Low-back pain is more common, is usually more serious, and deserves more attention. Herniated disks are rarely a problem in the upper back or thoracic spine, for example, while a herniated disk in the lower back or lumbar spine can pinch spinal nerves and cause weakness and loss of sensation in the legs or encroach upon the spinal canal to impair bladder or bowel function (cauda equina syndrome). This is why the Agency for Health Care Policy and Research (AHCPR) guidelines for treating low-back pain caution against manipulating the lumbar spine when there is leg pain caused by nerve-root involvement (see Appendix C).

Except when the thoracic vertebrae have been softened by disease or by aging, appropriate thoracic spine manipulation is rarely harmful and often can relieve backache related to fatigue, postural strain, arthritis, myofascitis, or other problems involving muscles and joints. Many people undergo thoracic spine manipulation simply for the relaxing effect that results from "popping the back."

Other Joints and Muscles

Uncomplicated mechanical-type problems of the muscles or joints of the shoulder, elbow, wrist, knee, ankle, and foot can often be helped by a competent chiropractor who uses physical therapy. Most chiropractors learn manipulative techniques for treatment of extremity joints, but these joints often benefit as much from mobilization as from manipulation. And they are often best treated by a physical therapist or an orthopedist. While chiropractors who have additional postgraduate training in orthopedics or sports medicine can be expected to have more extensive knowledge of injuries involving the extremities, none of them can prescribe pain medication, reduce a dislocated joint, set a broken bone, drain a swollen knee, or perform injections or invasive diagnostic procedures. Thus, a chiropractor with a diplomate in orthopedics or sports medicine cannot do much more than a physical therapist (other than manipulate the spine) or the average chiropractor. Although some physical therapists are now manipulating the spine, most are using mobilization techniques.

Severe or prolonged problems with extremity joints should always be brought to the attention of an orthopedist. As with back pain, diagnosis is essential. When a condition under chiropractic care has not improved after two to four weeks, a specialist should be consulted for a second opinion. On the other hand, there are many situations where home care can be effective once the diagnosis has been made and acute symptoms have subsided. A rational chiropractor will be able to advise when cost-saving self-care can be substituted for office treatment. It is rarely necessary to continue any form of chiropractic office treatment month after month. Here are two more case histories that illustrate these points:

• Oscar B visited my office complaining of shoulder pain. Physical examination revealed a painful shoulder with restriction of movement only in certain directions. X-ray examination did not reveal any calcific deposits or arthritic formations, and bone structure was normal. The diagnosis was supraspinatus tendinitis, an inflammation of the tendon of a muscle that helps move the upper arm away from the body. Tendinitis is a stubborn condition that can take several months to recover from. I advised Oscar to have ultrasound treatments at my office over a two-week period, after which he could either have more or continue self-treatment at home. I also said that if his pain grew worse, I would refer him to an orthopedist who might recommend medication and possibly a shoulder injection. After two weeks, he felt considerably better, his shoulder motion had increased, and he decided to treat himself at home. I explained how to use an overhead pulley, range-of-motion exercises, and cold and hot packs at home. I also advised that if he had an acute attack of shoulder pain that cold packs could not relieve, he should see an orthopedist. Within a few months he was fully recovered.

• Bill D also complained of shoulder pain, but his shoulder movement was normal and painless. He described the pain as deep and relentless, which had been tormenting him for months. When an x-ray examination of his shoulder and lung on the side of the pain revealed a large cancerous mass in the upper lobe of the lung, I immediately referred him to a physician.

Pain in other joints is not often as ominous as shoulder pain that might occur as a result of a problem with the heart or the lungs or because of a disk herniation in the neck. But it is always necessary to rule out bone tumors, advanced forms of arthritis, and other problems before beginning long-course treatment of any kind.

Tips on Choosing a Chiropractor

If you decide to consult a chiropractor, try to find one whose practice is limited to conservative treatment of musculoskeletal problems. Ask your family doctor for the names of chiropractors who fit this description and who appear to be competent and trustworthy. If your doctor cannot provide a name, ask other people and, if they recommend one, be sure to ask them

Chirobase Referral Directory Guidelines

My practice is limited to the care of musculoskeletal problems. My approach to back pain parallels the AHCPR Clinical Practice Guidelines that lie within the scope of chiropractic. I publicly endorse immunization, fluoridation, and other standard public health measures.

I reject biotheistic notions that "subluxations" and/or "nerve interference" are the cause or underlying cause of disease. I do not make claims about curing diseases. I do not try to get patients to sign contracts for lengthy treatment, promote regular "preventive" adjustments, use scare tactics, or disparage scientific medical treatment. I do not routinely perform or order x-ray examinations because most patients do not need them. I do not utilize 14" x 36" full-spine x-ray examinations.

I do not offer Biological Terrain Assessment, computerized "nutrient deficiency" testing, contact reflex analysis, contour analysis (also called moire contourography), cytotoxic testing, other improper allergy testing, electrodermal screening, Functional Intracellular Analysis (FIA), hair analysis, herbal crystallization analysis, iridology, leg-length testing, live blood cell analysis (also called nutritional blood analysis or Hemaview), testing with a Nervo-Scope, Nutrabalance, NUTRI-SPEC, pendulum divination, reflexology, saliva testing, spinal ultrasound testing to "measure progress," surface electromyography (SEMG), thermography, testing with a Toftness device, weighing on a twin-scale device (Spinal Analysis Machine), or any other diagnostic procedure that is unsubstantiated and lacks a scientifically plausible rationale.

I do not utilize acupuncture, Activator Methods, applied kinesiology, Bio Energetic Synchronization Technique (B.E.S.T.), chelation therapy, colonic irrigation, cranial or craniosacral therapy, laser acupuncture, magnetic or biomagnetic therapy, Neuro Emotional Technique (NET), Neural Organization Technique (N.O.T.), or any other treatment modality that is unsubstantiated and lacks a scientifically plausible rationale. I do not "prescribe" homeopathic products. I do not sell or promote the use of unproven dietary supplements or herbal products for the treatment of disease.

what conditions the chiropractor treats. If the chiropractor claims to treat infections or a wide range of other diseases, look elsewhere. But don't depend upon the Yellow Pages. You should avoid chiropractors who make extravagant claims, advertise extensively, or offer free examinations or consultations.

When you have selected a chiropractor, go for a consultation or conduct a telephone interview to find out how he or she practices. If the chiropractor treats infants, offers spinal adjustments as a treatment for visceral disease or infection or as a method of preventing ill health, requires that every patient be x-rayed, or requires payments in advance for a long course of treatments, call another chiropractor. The guidelines on the opposite page provide additional tips about what to avoid. Chiropractors who follow these guidelines have been invited to post their names in the referral directory on Chirobase, a Web site (http://www.chirobase.org) co-hosted by Stephen Barrett, M.D., editor of this book. Membership in the National Association for Chiropractic Medicine (NACM) (http://www.chiromed.org) is another favorable sign. NACM's application requires a written pledge to "openly renounce the historical chiropractic philosophical concept that subluxation is the cause of disease" and to limit their practice to nonsurgical musculoskeletal conditions.

Remember that diagnosis is critical to the establishment of proper treatment. Some chiropractors are competent in diagnosis, and some are not. For example, "straight" chiropractors who examine only the spine and who believe that "subluxated" vertebrae are the primary cause of illness may "analyze" the spine rather than offer a diagnosis. Such chiropractors may be unable to determine when chiropractic treatment should *not* be used. Since evaluating some chiropractors may be difficult, it might be wise to look for one who is willing to work with your family physician by exchanging office notes. This would offer the additional safeguard of assuring a second opinion.

Once you have found a rational chiropractor, you may find effective relief for some types of back and neck pain, as well as for various other musculoskeletal problems. You may also benefit from the comforting effect of a hands-on treatment that provides a pleasurable way of relieving the aches and pains of everyday stress and strain. Physical therapists, osteopaths, and a few physicians also offer manipulative therapy. Chiropractors can sometimes be found working with these practitioners in back-pain clinics. As the benefits of spinal manipulation become better known as a result of scientific research, such treatment will become more available from physical therapists and other practitioners, as well as from properly limited chiropractors.

14

Chiropractic Responses to My Criticisms

Reform-minded chiropractors are poorly tolerated by the chiropractic profession and may be ostracized if they speak out. Most chiropractors base their treatment on correcting the "vertebral subluxation complex" and regard any criticism as a threat to their livelihood. Many fear that because chiropractic owes its existence to subluxation theory, the profession cannot afford to tolerate criticism from within. Any pronouncement that spinal adjustments do not benefit general health is considered an attack on the entire profession. These cultist attitudes make conservative chiropractors reluctant to speak out. Most who do are denounced as traitors [86]. This chapter describes the various ways I have attempted to foster reform and the responses I have received from my colleagues.

My Early Skepticism

I have always been inclined to question things and to demand proof. Chapter 1 describes how I gradually diverged from mainstream chiropractic thinking during my chiropractic college years. In 1956, the year I graduated, most chiropractors offered chiropractic adjustments for the gamut of human ailments. People flocked to those who promised miracles but paid little attention to those who did not.

With a small practice and much time on my hands, I wrote a 291-page book called *Bonesetting, Chiropractic, and Cultism*, which was published in 1963. The book supported the appropriate use of spinal manipulation but renounced chiropractic dogma. It concluded:

159

The main trouble with chiropractic is chiropractic itself. Whatever might be correct in the use of manipulation is obviously not pursued by chiropractors. Furthermore, there do not seem to be any authorities within the realm of chiropractic with enough influence to successfully unite the various factions in chiropractic on factual and common grounds.

Establishment of chiropractic as a science would, of necessity, demand that chiropractors themselves clean and unite their own organization according to facts and standards characteristic of any recognized science in the healing arts, even if it meant rejection of a great deal of what has been known as chiropractic. [80]

Not long afterward, I received this notice from the American Chiropractic Association (ACA):

In regard to your recent application for membership in the American Chiropractic Association and insurance in the National Chiropractic Insurance Company, please be advised that the ACA membership committee has rejected your application. We are returning your checks in the amounts of $25.00 and $10.00 to you.

We are sorry we cannot be of service to you in this connection. [147]

Bonesetting, Chiropractic, and Cultism received a favorable review in the February 1, 1964, issue of the *Library Journal* [125], and a Stanford Research Institute official called it "most intriguing and enlightening" [154]. I received only negative responses from chiropractors. Discouraged by my apparent inability to communicate with my colleagues, I simply withdrew and concentrated on caring for my patients. But I continued to feel compelled to offer any criticism that might stimulate reform.

Further Efforts to Communicate

In 1983, I spoke out again in an article called "Chiropractic and Your Back" in *Muscular Development* magazine. I warned:

Many chiropractors still base their practice on the theory that most diseases can be treated by manipulating the vertebrae to relieve "nerve interference." . . . While chiropractors might be skillful in the performance of manipulation, not all of them will always place proper limitations upon its use. . . . So even if your chiropractor does a good job taking care of your back trouble and other neuromusculoskeletal problems, that doesn't mean that the same treatment will be effective in curing or preventing disease and infection. [81]

The ACA director of professional relations responded, in part: "Doctor Homola's tautological article on chiropractic and back problems sounds like many we have read lately by nonparticipators in the profession" [178].

In 1984, I submitted a critique entitled "This I Believe: Solving the Problems of Chiropractic" to the *Digest of Chiropractic Economics*. The associate editor returned the article with these comments:

> Our editorial board has reviewed this article and has declined the offer to publish it in our magazine. While it presents some well-defined arguments, its condemnation of the chiropractic profession is too far-reaching and that could pose many problems. We might find ourselves having to print a number of rebuttals stemming out of this one article. [189]

In 1991, in a letter inviting me to rejoin the ACA, its board chairman wrote:

> I enjoyed reading a copy of your article that appeared in the June 1983 issue of MUSCULAR DEVELOPMENT. The ACA must have been in the "Dark Ages" if they could not appreciate that article. However, it is consistent with the thinking of the current ACA leadership. [150]

That same year, I submitted an article entitled "Sense and Nonsense in Chiropractic Care of Back Pain" to *Dynamic Chiropractic*, the chiropractic profession's most widely read publication. It received a form-letter rejection.

In 1995, I wrote a similar article called "Sense and Nonsense in Chiropractic Care of the Back" for *Scholastic Coach* magazine [85]. While a few chiropractors agreed with my views, most criticized me severely. In personal correspondence, the executive director of the ACA Council on Sports Injuries and Physical Fitness wrote:

> Why did you find it necessary to address information contained within your article publicly? Why do you think chiropractors who can relieve a back pain cannot be trusted to treat any other kind of pain, regardless of what qualifications or specializations the chiropractor might have? I am sure you are familiar with the various councils of the ACA. Many chiropractors choose to continue their education in chiropractic through many methods. These specializations range from orthopedics, rehabilitation, internal diagnosis, radiology, nutrition, and neurology to sports injuries. . . . I can also refer you to several studies addressing the role of manipulation in some organic disease. . . . There are studies to support the response of the body's immune system with spinal manipulation. . . .

Unfortunately, this letter is probably nothing more than an exercise in futility. . . . If you don't intend to help the profession with your retoric [sic], why write? [89]

Letters in the August 1995 issue of *The Chiropractic Journal* (a subluxation-based newspaper) were much stronger [149]. One said my comments "will set chiropractic back 100 years." Another said, "Chiropractic is what it is. If you don't agree with its premise, please leave and do something else. You are a disgrace to chiropractic." A third one suggested that the Florida state board of chiropractic should reprimand me. Yet another said:

Samuel Homola is not a chiropractor but a chiropractoid. He deprives his patients, if he has any, of the benefits of chiropractic care and what it is capable of letting the body do—allowing it to obtain its individual optimum potential .

I was also attacked in a mass mailing with the salutation "Dear Colleague":

As we prepare to embrace this most commemorative year of Chiropractic, celebrating 100 years of our beloved profession, we still have a cancerous personality or two in our own profession who would like nothing more than to self-anoint themselves with recognition by exploiting their controversial viewpoint at the expense of the entire chiropractic profession. An individual who calls himself a chiropractor, Dr. Sam Homola, has just recently authored an article in the March, 1995 *Scholastic Coach and Athletic Director* publication. . . . This magazine has a widespread influence upon adults who serve as role models (coaches) for the young men and women who are aspiring to better their athletic ability and possibly become tomorrow's Olympians and super-stars. Obviously, this is an inappropriate forum for a chiropractor to assert his anti-chiropractic vantage point of our profession. . . . I believe this Chiropractor is more harmful to our profession today than he was 30 years ago. I would appreciate any insight that you may have. Please contact me personally . . . . if you feel this is worthy of any concern with respect to the future of the chiropractic profession. [172]

Obviously, few chiropractors would want to express a dissenting opinion if it means alienating from their colleagues. Chiropractic reformers who are active in their efforts to help place proper limitations upon chiropractic have to be prepared to withstand animosity that can be disturbing and threatening.

Chiropractic Journal Exposure

My views have also found little support in chiropractic journals. In 1992, *Chiropractic Technique* published my article called "Seeking a Common Denominator in the Use of Spinal Manipulation," which stated:

> Chiropractors make a unique and important contribution in their use of spinal manipulation as a method of treating neck and back trouble. The chiropractic profession as a whole remains largely unsupported by the scientific community, however, because of claims that spinal manipulation is effective in restoring and maintaining health. The theory supporting these claims has allowed the development of many unscientific practices among chiropractors. Proper limitations placed upon the use of spinal manipulation and a change in the definition of chiropractic would reduce exploitation of spinal manipulation and make the use of manipulation more available to referring physicians. This commentary is not a scientific treatise, but is simply an opinion based on observations made by the author. [84]

Subsequent letters to the editor came from three chiropractic colleges and a Canadian chiropractor. The administrative assistant to the president of Palmer College of Chiropractic wrote:

> To conform to such an idea would be to deny the very foundation of chiropractic.
> Chiropractic is based on the fundamental principle that homeostasis provides for the human body to self-repair provided there is no interference to the process. It is, therefore, logical that if the nerve flow to any organ of the body is interrupted, that organ will not be able to function at its optimum level. If nerve interference is removed and normal nerve impulses are permitted to flow again, the self-reparative mechanisms will be able to complete their task. [14]

The president of National College of Chiropractic agreed that slightly misaligned vertebrae are not likely to be harmful to health. But he felt that spinal adjustments have a beneficial effect on health:

> I have found, as have many others, that all too frequently there is an effect upon the human organism that results from spinal manipulation that is apart from the direct effects upon the somatic component which is being manipulated. . . . I certainly would not agree with Dr. Homola that the profession of chiropractic should restrict itself to the care of mechanical-type neuromusculoskeletal

problems and related elements. . . . And while I recognize Dr. Homola's right to express his opinion and I salute him for taking the time to do so, I, also, wish to clearly state my disagreement with his position. [202]

The Canadian chiropractor was more vehement:

All we ask is one thing, if you are calling yourself a chiropractor but don't believe, go practice under some other name or guise. Don't denounce, defame, or help to abolish our precious profession. We have to be different to survive. Our philosophy is what makes us different. We have a big enough job to do without resistance from within. It is our right to practice chiropractic the way it was and is meant to be. For the sake of humankind, let us allow them the opportunity to choose what is right. There are too many lives to be saved. [92]

The only favorable response came from an associate professor at Northwestern College of Chiropractic:

I was delighted and surprised by Dr. Samuel Homola's commentary. . . . Delighted, because of the rare insight and common sense demonstrated in his paper (i.e., he agrees with me). Surprised, because of the relative infrequency with which those qualities, insight and common sense, occur in the debate over chiropractic scope of practice. Bravo! Dr. Homola.

The irony is that the solution Dr. Homola prescribes, defining chiropractors as neuromusculoskeletal specialists, is the de facto scope of practice for the profession. All that remains is for chiropractors to embrace this state of affairs. Inexplicably, we are loath to do so. [128]

In 1995, on the heels of chiropractic's centennial celebration, *Chiropractic Technique* published an article in which I advised:

It is time to put aside support for the chiropractic subluxation theory and the philosophy supporting claims that "chiropractic works" for the gamut of human ailments for some reason not apparent to medical scientists. It is time to back away from contentions that spinal manipulation might be an effective treatment for renal colic, dysmenorrhea, ear infection, and similar ailments.

If the chiropractic profession concentrated the bulk of its research on physical treatment for mechanical-type neck and back problems, everything else would take care of itself. [82]

The executive director of the Foundation for Chiropractic Education and Research (FCER) replied:

I have no doubt that Dr. Samuel Homola's article . . . was well intentioned. However, it exhibited a lack of documentation and his conclusions were based largely on conjecture and speculation. Unfortunately, although some of Dr. Homola's opinions are flawed but benign, others could threaten the future of the chiropractic profession. . . . It has long been the contention of FCER that to position chiropractors as "back doctors" would be disastrous for the future of the profession and would only serve to limit the choice of treatments available to patients. Based on substantial anecdotal evidence supporting chiropractic intervention, FCER is funding research that investigates chiropractic treatment for the very ailments that Dr. Homola recommends that we back away from: colic, dysmenorrhea, and ear infection. [161]

Think about this for a moment. Is chiropractic's foundation so tenuous that the entire profession could be toppled by a single opinion?

Contact with the Medical Profession

In 1998, my article "Finding a Good Chiropractor" was published in the AMA's *Archives of Family Medicine.* Its abstract offered this advice to physicians:

Spinal manipulation provided by chiropractors is often beneficial in the treatment of some types of back pain. Since some chiropractors use spinal manipulation to treat visceral disease and back pain, medical practitioners may have to be cautious and selective in referring patients with back pain to chiropractors. This commentary will help family physicians determine when it might be appropriate to seek the services of a chiropractor in the treatment of back pain. [83]

To my knowledge, this was the first article written by an individual chiropractor ever published in an AMA journal. You might think that chiropractic editors would find this event newsworthy. To date, however, this article has not been mentioned in any chiropractic publication I have seen. I can only assume that the profession continues to discourage dissemination of views that denounce subluxation theory.

Reform Will Not Come Easily

Based on my own experience, I have concluded that subluxation theory is still deeply entrenched among members of my profession. Until chiropractic colleges and major organizations stop pretending that subluxations are an underlying cause of ill health, few chiropractors will be inclined or able to dispute what they have been taught. And those who do will continue to be criticized by those who are economically and philosophically committed. The next and final chapter outlines what I believe chiropractic must do to secure a legitimate place in the healthcare marketplace.

15

Is Reform
Likely?

When I graduated from chiropractic college in 1956, I saw no reason to believe that chiropractic adjustments had any legitimate role in treating disease. But I felt that appropriate spinal manipulation was valuable for treating mechanical-type musculoskeletal problems. After forty-three years of practice, I still feel the same way.

Throughout my career, I made a special effort to select cases that I felt were appropriate for the limited treatment methods I employed. Without directly criticizing my chiropractic colleagues, I also discouraged patients from seeking inappropriate chiropractic care. And since appropriate manipulation was not readily available elsewhere—even from most chiropractors—I found that my services were well appreciated by patients and by the local medical community.

It is not easy to disagree with my colleagues, and it is painful to generate discomfort and animosity among my many chiropractic friends. But critical analysis is needed—both to protect the public and to encourage further development of spinal manipulation as science.

Some observers believe that chiropractic will evolve into a limited specialty, since it cannot or should not continue to define itself as a method of correcting spinal problems to restore and maintain health. In *Chiropractic: History and Evolution of a New Profession*, Walter Wardwell, Ph.D., drew these conclusions about chiropractic's future:

> My overall conclusions are that the role of chiropractic in the U.S. health care system will continue to change, that chiropractors will

167

probably not remain in as marginal a social and professional role as they have known for nearly a century, that they will not track osteopaths into the medical mainstream, and that they will most likely evolve slowly into a "limited medical" status comparable to that of dentists, podiatrists, optometrists, and psychologists. [191]

At this point, it is not clear to me that the chiropractic profession is making the changes needed to develop into a properly limited specialty. Efforts by leaders in the profession to define chiropractic as an "alternative" healing method align it with faddish practices that will eventually lose the support of an informed public. If the chiropractic profession is to change course in the future, many things must be done.

Subluxation Nonsense Must Be Abandoned

As noted in Chapter 4, chiropractors define subluxations in many ways and cannot agree about what they are, how they should be diagnosed, how they should be treated, or even what they should be called. Some consider subluxations to be physical or physiologic entities, while others assign metaphysical attributes. The resultant confusion has alienated other professionals as well as policy-makers who control access to patients who could benefit from rational chiropractic care.

Although most patients who consult chiropractors have musculoskeletal problems, subluxation theory encourages chiropractors to believe that their scope is unlimited and that they should be considered primary care practitioners [39,75]. However, the prevailing definition of primary care is "the provision of integrated, accessible health care services by clinicians who are accountable for addressing a large majority of personal health needs . . ." [44]. Chiropractors do not fit this definition.

In my opinion, unless chiropractors abandon subluxation theory and properly limit their scope, they will remain marginalized. The National Association for Chiropractic Medicine requires renunciation of subluxation dogma as a condition of membership, but they are a small group and have little impact on the profession as a whole.

Appropriate Research Is Needed

Chiropractic research has yet to pinpoint what chiropractors do that is beneficial. Although the RAND and AHCPR panels have concluded that spinal manipulation is useful for treating certain types of back pain, their conclusions were based primarily on research—done mainly by physicians and physical therapists—that does not necessarily reflect what chiropractors do in their offices.

To gain scientific acceptance, chiropractors will have to do much more research—not only to establish what might work, but also to establish what does *not* work. However, chiropractic interest in doing this does not appear to be high. In 1996, a questionnaire on research priorities was mailed to 2,280 chiropractors, of which 1,245 responded. The researchers concluded:

> The very lowest rated objective, with only 3% of the respondents choosing it, was *increasing the ability of the profession to conduct its own research.* . . .
>
> Of the choices presented to them in this study, American chiropractors are less interested in research which develops or evaluates chiropractic techniques, procedures, and equipment, which helps to establish practice parameters, or which improves the effectiveness of chiropractic education, and are least interested in that which increases the ability of the profession to conduct its own research.
>
> Practicing chiropractors in the United States feel that the *acceptance of chiropractic, primarily by patients and other health care professionals*, is the most important research objective. . . . However, it is curious that they feel that this can be best and most immediately accomplished by means of basic science research on the nature of the subluxation complex and/or the physiological effects of adjustments, including visceral and neuromusculoskeletal effects. [94]

Tight Guidelines Are Needed

Many organizations and agencies establish expert panels that review scientific reports and develop evidence-based clinical practice guidelines that are highly respected by the scientific medical community. The recently established National Guidelines Clearinghouse has catalogued hundreds of them. Although chiropractors held a major consensus conference in 1992, the resultant document is relatively vague, has not been widely accepted by chiropractors, and has done little to alter how they treat patients (see Chapter 3).

Even worse, the profession as a whole has done almost nothing to confront its rampant quackery. Although a few methods have been debunked by studies published in chiropractic journals, these studies appear to have little or no influence on what chiropractors do.

Educational Reform Is Needed

With few exceptions, chiropractic colleges still teach subluxation theory and permit philosophy to overshadow science. While some students acquire sufficient skill to manage various musculoskeletal problems, others emerge with an affinity for nonsense. Joseph Keating, Ph.D., a research expert who has taught at several chiropractic colleges, recently warned:

> Many of the schools are magnets for New Agers, theosophists, magical and mystical thinkers, and those attracted by the low admissions standards and the lure of a lucrative private practice.... Moreover, since the largest chiropractic colleges tend to have the strongest commitments to dogma, fuzzy thinkers are likely to fill the chiropractic ranks for decades to come. [101]

The Council on Chiropractic Education (CCE), which accredits the schools, not only has lax standards but also fails to ensure that they are properly met. Solving this problem will require a major overhaul of CCE's activities and probably cannot be done unless the council is reconstituted to include reform-minded critics. The U.S. Secretary of Education should seriously consider rescinding CCE's approved status unless a radical change takes place. The "straight" chiropractic colleges that are immersed in Palmerian dogma probably cannot be reformed.

Anyone considering a chiropractic career should investigate very carefully. I believe that more chiropractors are graduating than the market-place can absorb and that this situation will worsen as time goes on. (It has been estimated that by 2010 there will be 103,000 chiropractors, about 70% more than today) [48]. Although the failure rate is unknown, chiropractors have by far the highest student loan default rate among those who attend health-related professional schools. As of mid-1998, 817 of 1,495 defaulters were chiropractors who owed an average of $72,200 each.

Dangers Must Be Confronted

Although chiropractors insist that the incidence of stroke and other serious complications of cervical manipulation is low, no effort has been made to gather and publish meaningful data. I believe that chiropractic organizations should set up a registry and an investigative body to determine, once and for all, how often complications occur and under what circumstances. Many observers believe that extreme rotation with hyperextension of the neck is a major factor and should be abandoned. Chiropractic organizations should examine this and develop a position paper on this subject.

Public Health Measures Must Be Endorsed

As noted in Chapter 3, many chiropractors are either opposed to immunization procedures or feel that they should be voluntary rather than compulsory. Many chiropractic colleges foster similar beliefs. The International Chiropractors Association (ICA) and other straight organizations oppose immunization, while the American Chiropractic Association (ACA) is lukewarm. The ICA also opposes water fluoridation, while the ACA has ignored the issue. Chiropractors and their organizations should join the rest of the scientific community in unequivocally endorsing immunization and fluoridation. Chiropractic colleges should advocate them, and the Council on Chiropractic Education should insist on this as a condition for accreditation.

Is Reform Likely?

The most embarrassing criticism chiropractic has ever received took place on February 4, 1994, when ABC-TV's *20/20* described visits to seventeen chiropractors who treated children. The visits were videotaped so there could be no doubt about the program's accuracy.

One segment showed what happened when nine New York chiropractors examined an infant with recurring ear infections, a problem that a pediatrician had said was manageable with antibiotics and would eventually be outgrown. Another segment described how eight Wisconsin chiropractors responded to a five-year-old boy with chronic ear infections so severe that medical doctors wanted to insert tubes in his ears to drain them. Each of the chiropractors found at least one problem, but nearly all disagreed about its nature and location. All said they could help and recommended care ranging from several weeks to a lifetime. Their diagnostic procedures and conclusions were patently ridiculous. For example, two diagnosed the infant's problem by testing the strength of *his mother's* arm or leg ("surrogate testing"), and two diagnosed unequal leg lengths in the five-year-old but differed about which one was shorter.

In another segment, Larry Webster, D.C., the leading promoter of "chiropractic pediatrics" claimed he had cured a child's deafness in two visits and would provide the family's telephone number. Off camera, however, he said he couldn't locate it. In another segment, the mother of one of Webster's patients said proudly that her child had not been immunized, and another mother described how Webster had cured her child's ear infection with manipulation.

The March 1994 *ACA Journal of Chiropractic* devoted fifteen pages to the "20/20 incident." Former ACA board chairman Louis Sportelli, D.C., editorialized:

> Hasn't this profession been harmed enough by proclaiming cures and peddling techniques which have never been validated? Hasn't the image of this profession been tarnished enough in lawsuits and headline after headline? When are we going to say *enough is enough*? When is the New York Board of Chiropractic Examiners, and other boards across this country, going to look at these aberrant practices and demand validation or at least some proof that some scientific process is currently under way to substantiate the procedures claimed? . . .
>
> The program clearly identified the kind of chiropractic practice which is unacceptable to most of the chiropractic community and certainly to the consuming public. It identified the type of practitioner and the type of gimmicks of which the consumer should beware. . . .
>
> In my opinion, it was the actions of a few practitioners that caused this professional disgrace, doctors who use mystical and magical methods on tiny tots without reasonable protocols or rational treatment methods. Infants and children deserve chiropractic without a doubt, but they deserve a competent evaluation, a reasonable examination, an honest appraisal, and a fair, but limited, trial of chiropractic care by a competent practitioner using defensible procedures taught in accredited chiropractic colleges. What they do not deserve is gimmicks to entice them, shoddy procedures to examine them, unreasonable treatment given to them and false hope to hold them. [181]

Will chiropractic colleges, licensing boards, or prominent organizations ever declare war on the gimmicks, shoddy examination procedures, unreasonable treatments, or promotion of false hopes that are documented throughout this book? Will chiropractic leaders ever admit that chiropractic "aberrations" are not the exception but the rule? Can chiropractic's absurd procedures disappear without abandonment of metaphysical "subluxation" concepts? Will chiropractic ever define its appropriate scope? Will research ever pinpoint what chiropractors do that is helpful? Is there reason to believe that chiropractic can be reformed?

I, myself, am not optimistic. Unless and until major improvements take place, if you decide to see a chiropractor, choose carefully!

Appendix A

A Scientific Brief
Against Chiropractic (1963)

This report was excerpted from the Brief of the College of Physicians and Surgeons of the Province of Quebec submitted in 1963 to the Royal Commission on Chiropractic, which was appointed by the Quebec legislature to study the chiropractic question and make recommendations on the advisability of licensing chiropractors in the province. The college prepared the brief in an effort to persuade the Royal Commission that the licensing of chiropractors in Quebec was not in the best interests of the public health. This excerpt was originally published in the September 1966 issue of *The New Physician*, the journal of the Student American Medical Association. It presents an exceptionally well-reasoned analysis of the fallacies of subluxation theory.

Introduction

The present century has been called the age of the scientific revolution. The advantage to contemporary man is enormous not only because of the everyday practical application of these discoveries, but also because he has thrown off the yoke of superstition. In this era of superhuman achievements, each intelligent individual owes it to himself to apply scientific criteria before accepting any new theory of nature's phenomena.

The foundation of scientific method is experimentation. Nothing can be accepted as fact, no relationship between two facts can be accepted as established unless experimentation has proved it beyond all doubt. The scientist must construct his experiment in such a way as to not only establish each fact he is seeking, but also to prove that no other explanation is possible. He must build a tight network of proof and counterproof until no possibility of error in judgment remains before allowing himself the certainty that he has achieved an element of truth. The laws of nature transcend those of man, and one must bow to them or risk lamentable errors and their inexorable consequences.

Chiropractic was invented not long after the discoveries of Pasteur in chemistry and bacteriology and of Claude Bernard in physiology; at the same time as those of Pavlov on conditioned reflexes, of Crookes on cathode rays, of Hertz on TSF waves, of Roentgen on x-rays, and of Becquerel on radioactivity. It was precisely in 1895 that Jean Perrin completed the experimental concept of electrons after Lorentz, Zeeman, Thompson, Millikan, and Wilson had progressively defined their properties.

The list of discoveries which were contemporary to the invention of chiropractic and which inaugurated the age of the scientific revolution could be extended almost indefinitely. It was the time of the extraordinary work of the Curies, which paved the way for the development of atomic energy. It must not, of course, be held against D.D. Palmer that he was not a scientific scholar, nor should anyone be denied the opportunity of making a scientific observation. But before accepting the reliability of that observation, or drawing conclusions from it, and above all before applying any theory derived from it to the treatment of human ills, we have the right and indeed the responsibility to submit it to at least the minimum exigencies of scientific proof.

This duty devolves primarily on those who profess the chiropractic theory. Chiropractors have had every scientific method available to them. Sixty-eight years constitute a sufficient period for the experimental proof of a limited number of facts. Such experimental proof should be prerequisite to the application in practice of such a theory. What experimental proof has been furnished by the chiropractor?

Lack of Scientific Support for Chiropractic Theory

Perturbation of the Distribution of Nervous Impulses
Chiropractors claim that subluxations, or partial displacements, of the vertebrae cause a perturbation of the distribution of nervous impulses to tissues and cells. Neurophysiologists have developed methods of recording the passage of impulses in nerves. Exceptionally sensitive apparatus is

available to anyone wishing to use it. No scientific study has been published on the subject by a chiropractor. No chiropractor has ever defined, either quantitatively or qualitatively, what chiropractic means by perturbation of nervous impulses. Is it their number, their amplitude, their frequency, the speed of their propagation, or their wave patterns which are affected? All of these qualities can be identified, recorded, and studied. It is no longer permissible to accept empirical statements. Proof should have preceded practical application. With the first point untenable, the rest crumbles. In pure scientific logic, the argument should not need to go farther than this.

Perturbation of Health and Determination of Illness

Chiropractors affirm that alterations in the distribution of nervous impulses to tissues and cells disturb the state of health and provoke the illnesses which they treat. By what experimental proof have they demonstrated a causative relationship between disturbances of nervous flow and the development of illnesses which they claim to cure? Here, again, absolutely none. The defectiveness of this link in this chain, added to the defectiveness of the first, increases, if that be possible, the fallacy of the whole.

It is indeed astonishing that there has been such a lack of effort, or of concern for scientific truth, especially if one considers the effort which has gone into selling the theory to the general public—when the world to be convinced was the scientific world. Let the theory gain acceptance in the world of scholars, and all the troubles of the chiropractor will vanish.

The Localization of Obstructions

Once again, chiropractors affirm that their technique enables them to detect and localize "obstructions which, in the mechanics of the human body, alter the distribution and physiologic action of nervous impulses." They explain that in most cases these anatomic modifications are barely beyond the limits of the physiologic state. It seems reasonable that generations of men over the past 68 years would have accumulated data and developed increasingly accurate and sensitive methods of measuring and recording.

It should also be pointed out that anyone, chiropractor or layman, can buy an x-ray machine, since no law restricts the sale or use of such apparatus. Chiropractors have therefore been at liberty to use x-ray pictures and fluoroscopy in their studies. It should also be pointed out that many challenging diseases occur in the region of the vertebral column, and anyone who regularly examines this region must undoubtedly become reasonably skilled in recognizing deviations from normal which might be shown in malpositions of vertebrae, localized pains, spasms, muscular atrophies, bone spurs, inflammatory nodules, limitations of movement, etc. Every such person should be able, by means of these observations, to pinpoint the site in the vertebral column of the pathological process.

Therefore, it seems necessary to cast grave doubt on the diagnostic reliability of chiropractic examinations, if one considers that in many more serious and more extensive diseases of the vertebral column it is necessary to inject into the spinal canal a substance opaque to x-rays (a technique which chiropractors do not use) so that a highly trained specialist may achieve an accurate diagnosis of the location of the pathologic process. Chiropractors, with lesser means, claim a greater precision of diagnosis. But here again, no scientific proof supports the claim.

The Use of X-rays by Chiropractors: "Spinography"
One might think that chiropractors taking x-ray pictures could derive as much information from them as anyone else, and thus achieve a radiologic diagnosis as precise and accurate as that of a medical radiologist. The chiropractor generally purchases x-ray apparatus and uses it in a way which is termed Spinography or radiography of the spine. However, chiropractors are prone to exceed the limits of their competence and to obtain x-ray images of many various organs—in the interpretation of which they are handicapped by their lack of the lengthy and specialized training which is indispensable for the proper evaluation and interpretation of structures as seen on film.

A casual survey reveals that only about ten percent of the chiropractors of the Province of Quebec do not have x-ray apparatus. The 90% who do may be divided into two groups: Approximately two-thirds, or 60% of the total, use equipment adequate for authentic "Spinography." The remainder, about 30% of all chiropractors, use films of small dimension in apparatus of low intensity.

To the chiropractor, classical "Spinography" consists of a single picture, 36 inches high and 14 inches wide, of the entire vertebral column. This film is obtained with a very wide stream of radiation, which blankets almost the whole trunk of the body as it penetrates from the front to the film at the back. It is unusual for the chiropractor to take a side view, since the technical difficulties are great and the resulting film even less satisfactory than the antero-posterior view.*

—————————————

*Nowadays only about 15% of chiropractors in the United States and Canada use spinography, side views are commonly obtained, and the general quality of chiropractic x-ray films is much better.

Lines, traced in radio-opaque ink on one of the fluorescent screens inside the cassette which contains the film, superimpose on the spinographic picture a white graph, usually in two-inch squares. In theory, the purpose of these squares is to help visualize disturbances in the longitudinal alignment of the vertebral column. This technical detail does not really provide a better demonstration of possible changes in vertebral structure, external or internal; on the contrary, it may interfere with visibility.

Large films of this type, taken in the antero-posterior view only, have very limited diagnostic value. Ever since the earliest days of medical radiology, physicians have known the necessity of two views at right angles to one another—antero-posterior and lateral—because the antero-posterior view alone superimposes all structures, organs, and tissues in a two-dimensional picture. A view at right angles separates these superimposed elements and provides the third dimension. Thus the two views, front and side, are considered obligatory and are used systematically in medical radiology; even then, they are only an indispensable minimum and a first step to adequate x-ray evaluation. The side view in "Spinography," however, is quite rare. Even rarer in chiropractic are oblique views at a 45° angle, right and left—yet this is standard or even routine practice in medical radiology.

Over and above these techniques, where any uncertainty remains as to the existence, nature, or extent of a lesion, a whole series of special procedures is available to the medical radiologist for greater diagnostic precision—stereography, tomography, myelography, angiography, x-ray cinematography, etc, according to the case. These procedures, because of their complexity, often require the collaboration of various experts—orthopedists, neurologists, neurosurgeons, et al)—not only for their technical execution but also for the interpretation of the x-ray shadows and their correlation with the clinical findings.

These procedures were created and perfected to provide the closest possible approach to exact truth, and to allow the greatest possible precision in establishing the existence, the minute localization, and the veritable nature of any lesion.

It can be seen that these methods leave "Spinography" far behind, since, in addition to their rigorous technical requirements, they demand a truly profound knowledge of what is normal and what is not. In comparison with radiologic methods used by physicians in studying the vertebral column, "Spinography" in the chiropractic sense seems a very primitive technique, as likely to confuse as to inform, and able at best to provide gross information of limited reliability.

Even if pictures are taken at an adequate distance (six to eight feet) from x-ray tube to film, the curvatures (normal or abnormal) of the vertebral column cause some degree of superimposition of the shadows of adjacent vertebrae, the one on the other. The oblique direction of the x-rays in relation to these curvatures causes only certain vertebrae to be clearly distinguished from their neighbors above and below; and, indeed, focusing on a small area with careful aim is essential for the proper study of the outline and internal structure of each bone and of its relations to contiguous anatomical elements.

The difference in transparency between the air-filled thorax and the organ-filled abdomen, as well as differences in shape, thickness, and position between thoracic and lumbar vertebrae, cause a single film to show the thoracic vertebrae too darkly and the lumbar vertebrae too palely for proper diagnosis of their fine details of structure.

Radiologists accustomed to using large-scale films have devised compensatory screens to equalize the densities of thoracic and lumbar vertebrae in their pictures. Only rarely do chiropractors use these compensatory screens.

It is, therefore, because of the poor diagnostic quality of these oversize films that physicians reject their use for accurate evaluation of normal and abnormal conditions of the spine. Small sectional views are of much more diagnostic value than a single broad picture, since they provide a more accurate perspective of architectural relationships; they allow the photographic density to be adjusted for each region; and they require less scatter of x-rays, thereby giving a better quality of film and reducing the risk of genetic effects.

It may be estimated that about 30% of chiropractors use small films, but their reason for doing so is not the same as that of medical radiologists; rather, it is because their machines have insufficient power to take films at greater distance. They are therefore obliged to use longer exposure times, which impair the sharpness of detail. It is common to hear chiropractors affirm that:

(a) They see "subluxations" in their x-rays which radiologists, neurologists, orthopedists, rheumatologists, physiatrists, and others are unable to, or do not know how to see;

(b) The "subluxations" to which they refer are not the same as those defined in classical medical terms. (But words are words nonetheless, and to avoid the confusion of Babel it seems necessary to adhere to dictionary definitions and accepted usage.)

Chiropractic was officially born in 1895, the year in which Roentgen discovered x-rays. Although chiropractors originally claimed that their hands alone sufficed for the detection of the most minor defects of the spine, and for the relief of the supposed effects of the hypothetical pinching of spinal nerves, more and more of them have come to include the prestige of the x-ray machine in their arsenal of persuasion.

In all the years that they have been talking about them, chiropractors have never been able to furnish proof of these mysterious subluxations which they alone are able to see. They may convince their clients, but never—with or without "Spinography"—have they provided proof of their pretensions to men of science.

Furthermore, every physician knows that it suffices to have a patient bend slightly forward, or back, or to either side, to see evidences of movement—or, in other words, of displacements of articular surfaces one upon the other—in x-ray pictures. Such displacements are obviously phenomena of normal movement in the skeletal system, but when "stopped" in an x-ray photograph give an impression of permanence. In other words, the taker of the film may create, voluntarily or involuntarily, false "subluxations." A small error in the positioning of the patient's feet, for example, or in the alignment of his body at the instant of taking the picture, would be sufficient to give a false impression to an improperly trained person.

Long and repeated experience has taught orthopedists, radiologists, and indeed all physicians, that deviations of the spine, with displacements of articular surfaces of small or even large degree, and distortion of the intervertebral spaces where the disks are found, may result from a difference in the lengths of the two limbs, or from a tilt of the pelvis.

Abnormal curvatures of the spine, and malformations or malpositions of these elements of the skeleton, are often encountered on x-rays; they may be congenital, or due to disturbances of growth, or may even be sequelae of previous ailments (tuberculosis, poliomyelitis, cancer, injury, etc). Even in these cases, it must be remembered that spinal disturbances often accompany lower static disturbances—in the pelvis, the legs, or the feet; these latter may be the fundamental problem, and may therefore require correction before the vertebral column can be evaluated and treated.

In summary, "Spinography" is much more apt to deceive chiropractors and their clients than to prove the presence or absence of nerve pinching or the nature of the supposed compression.

However, the precision of radiologic information does not seem to be the chief aim of the chiropractor. Let us take, for example, what a teacher of chiropractic instructs his students on the value of "Spinography." In a book entitled *Modern X-Ray Practice and Chiropractic Spinography*, P. A. Remier, a member of the staff of the Palmer College of Chiropractic in Davenport, Iowa, devotes a short chapter to 50 "Reasons why the chiropractor should spinograph every case." From this list, one can select at least 13 reasons which seem to have little to do with science:

1. It promotes confidence.
2. The analysis could not be complete or correct without the spinograph.
3. It creates interest among patients.
4. It procures business.
5. It attracts a better class of patients.
6. It adds prestige in your community.
7. It builds a reliable reputation.
8. It is an investment and not an expense.
9. It provides good interest on your investment.
10. Its income makes it possible to arrange a better service.
11. It enables one to care for more patients daily.
12. It helps to eliminate the so-called starvation period that many practitioners go through.
13. It discloses the other fellow's mistakes.

It must be concluded that the manner in which chiropractors make use of x-rays demonstrates that they lack the necessary background in physics, biology, pathology, and clinical medicine to be able to use them effectively and safely on human beings. They may easily learn to operate an x-ray machine and to develop a film, but their deficiencies in basic knowledge, in equipment, and in technical training prevent them from turning out, consistently and safely, the documents necessary for the x-ray diagnosis of diseases or defects of the vertebral column, the craniospinal axis, or other organs or tissues.

The chiropractor's lack of medical background in radiology exposes him to letting serious illnesses pass unnoticed, or to giving unwarranted pathological significance to normal shadows. In other words, there is the Scylla of failing to see the disease which exists, and there is the Charybdis of thinking disease is present when actually it is not. There is also a temptation to exhibit the x-ray picture in order to impress the patient, and to beguile him into accepting chiropractic manipulation.

Over and above all this is the undeniable fact that "Spinography," i.e., the single x-ray of the whole spine on which chiropractors rely, has never demonstrated the pinching of a nerve, since nerves are not visible on x-ray films and can only be demonstrated by the injection of liquid or gaseous contrast media.

A further fact: After the age of 40, perfectly normal vertebral columns become rapidly rarer and rarer. It is unusual after that age to see spines without x-ray evidence of aging, including thinning of the disks and thinning and slipping of articular surfaces—but this in no way proves that nerves are pinched. The longer a man lives, the more impressive the radiologic changes in his vertebral column become.

Readjustment of the Vertebrae
Chiropractors claim to relieve obstructions by readjusting the vertebrae through manipulation. Once the vertebral column has been realigned, they instruct the patient in methods of preventing a recurrence. There is no denying that the vertebral column can be influenced by mechanical means; some means, however, have been shown to be quite dangerous. The issue revolves around the fact that no chiropractor has ever produced an original study of scientific value on the subject. There is surely no lack of scolioses, kyphoses, and lordoses—frank deviations of the vertebral column—in the population. It is astonishing to find that in precisely these conditions which might be dramatically helped if the manipulative technique were valid, chiropractors neither evince a special interest nor claim a special success.

One is forced to conclude that chiropractic has no scientific foundation. Invented empirically, it has developed in the same unbroken empiricism, taking no account of even the most minimal requirements of scientific proof. The same is true of its methods of application; it remains an unproven hypothesis which should not be risked in the treatment of ill persons.

Discussion of the Clinical Argument:
The Satisfied Customer

Nonetheless, chiropractors seem entirely satisfied with their theory, even though it has not changed since its invention, except for a few terms of nomenclature. They argue that even if their method is not scientifically proven, it is clinically. They mean by this that a legion of satisfied clients bear eloquent witness to their success. We freely admit that certain clients have been pleased with chiropractic treatment, and that some of them had previously consulted physicians and have preferred chiropractic treatment. The opposite is also true. This type of testimonial can readily be obtained on either side.

The same argument is invoked to assert that the public wants chiropractic, that it is no longer necessary to question the validity of the theory, that the public has judged. It may be permissible, however, to submit this point to the enlightened judgment of a Royal Commission.

The argument of the satisfied customer, which philosophers call the argument of "consensus universalis," falls in the category of moral certitude. In contrast to physical certitude—based on the immutable laws of nature, which scientific method provides, moral proof—based on the fallible and variable judgment of human beings according to their subjective impressions and previous experience—is necessarily of a much lower order, especially when applied to natural phenomena. To neglect physical certitude and fall back on moral proof is in itself a confession of the weakness of the argument.

Further, it would be necessary for that moral proof to be based on a unanimous consensus of uniform testimonials for its validity to be accepted. In the case in point, not all clients are satisfied with chiropractic; some who were satisfied at one time become dissatisfied later on. Further still, the quality of the proof depends on the quality of the testimony; and the quality of testimony is largely determined by the understanding which the witness has of the subject in question. To what degree can a person unaware of the nature and cause of his illness, and of chiropractic theory and the effects of chiropractic treatment, give valid evidence of a cause-and-effect relationship? It is surely unnecessary to emphasize to this Commission that thousands of unproven testimonials do not by sheer numbers constitute valid proof.

Indeed, it is well known that the patient's satisfaction is not always a reliable index of the value of the treatment he has received. Even if one were to overlook the fallacy of the moral proof and take it for granted for the sake of hypothesis, it would still be necessary to reject the argument. Disease is one of the phenomena of nature, and is therefore governed by natural laws; only by recognizing the laws of nature can one hope to cure disease. Any method of treatment which is not founded on the laws of nature is inevitably doomed to fail. To accept moral proof alone in the case of chiropractic would be to deny not only the existence of science but the order of nature as well.

One would nevertheless have to be blind to deny that chiropractors and their clients have increased in number. The explanation of this phenomenon would require a more extensive study than is possible here. Certain observations, however, would indicate where the sociologic reasons are to be found. In the early part of this century, up till the 1930s, physical medicine and rehabilitation had not received the attention of the medical profession, nor been given the importance they enjoy today. Nowadays the physiatrist, or physician specializing in physical medicine and rehabilitation, is certified in his specialty by the College of Physicians just as are surgeons, obstetricians, and gynecologists, et al.

During those years, medical efforts were directed towards more urgent tasks, such as the development of bacteriology, the struggle against contagious diseases, the evolution of precision and finesse in diagnosis, the enlargement and reinforcement of the therapeutic arsenal, the invention of techniques in surgery of the heart and brain, the improvement of therapy in mental illness, etc. In short, there were matters of greater urgency to be dealt with, conditions which are still found today in under-developed areas to an even more serious degree. Thus, chiropractic has seemed to offer hope in an area which medicine had appeared to overlook.

Since most people are very exacting of the physician, and therefore tend not to refer to any errors they may have made in consulting other persons but to get inordinate pleasure from any apparent success, failures do less harm to the chiropractor's reputation—especially since he can take refuge in the statement that the problem is not in his domain. But if the patient experiences a spontaneous cure while undergoing a series of chiropractic treatments, the value of the treatment is claimed to be nothing short of miraculous.

We shall see later on that there are indeed a small number of painful conditions of the spine which can be helped by manipulation. We must add forthwith that this does not mean that the chiropractic theory is valid, nor that chiropractic treatment is without danger. We shall see later that quite the opposite is true.

Having achieved considerable success against the scourges of the early part of the century, medicine turned to the development of physiatry, the objectives of which are not only the application of existing treatments, but their improvement and the discovery of more effective methods. At best, chiropractic could only hope to fill a role which medicine had not yet sufficiently developed. Nevertheless, it retains for certain people that mystic attraction which empirical and unaccepted theories and practices seem to have.

Scientific Evidence against Chiropractic

Chiropractic in Relation to Experimental Science
The fact that chiropractic is unsupported by any real scientific facts would alone be sufficient for its rejection as a method of treatment without further discussion. Nevertheless, it seems appropriate to examine the question objectively and consider the scientific disproof of the method.

In order to achieve a better understanding of the question, one must review as simply and clearly as possible certain concepts regarding the nervous system and the vertebral column. It is obvious that these few details cannot even approach a thorough survey of scientific knowledge on the subject.

The spinal nerves, which are the prime concern of chiropractic theory, extend from the vertebral column via the intervertebral foramina, which are short canals formed by the superimposition of pedicles jutting out from each vertebra. From the base of the skull to the pelvis, the vertebrae—7 cervical, 12 thoracic or dorsal, 5 lumbar, the sacrum, and the coccyx—form a long bony mast which supports the head above and stands on the pelvis (of which the sacrum and coccyx are actually part).

The sacrum and the coccyx are each a distinct bone. The sacrum is formed by the fusion of five sacral vertebrae into a single unit; the coccyx is a fusion of four to six rather rudimentary vertebrae. The cervical, dorsal, and lumbar vertebrae are all individual. The vertebrae have certain structural characteristics in common but also show certain regional differences in the various divisions of the vertebral column.

Each vertebra has a large cylindrical body anteriorly, with a bony arch extending backwards from it to form a circle; these circles, one above the other, form the spinal canal. On the bony arch, near its origin from the vertebral body on each side, there is a pedicle above and below. The vertebrae are so placed that each pedicle meets its neighbor, leaving between them and the vertebral bodies those orifices which are called intervertebral foramina. Through these foramina pass the spinal nerves.

Thus the vertebrae are aligned one above the other, vertebral body to vertebral body in front, and articular surface to articular surface on the arches behind. Between the vertebral bodies are disks which fill the spaces and are therefore called intervertebral disks. These disks resemble little cushions and are shaped like a biconvex lens. They are attached to the surfaces of the vertebral bodies above and below. They are relatively firm at their periphery, but soft and gelatinous in the center.

Finally, the bony arches of the vertebrae have two types of projection: one, called the spinous process, extends backwards from the arch in the midline (it is these spinous processes which are felt all down the back); the other, the transverse processes, extend laterally on each side from a position posterior to the intervertebral foramen.

If one now considers the vertebral column as a structural unit, one sees the column of vertebral bodies anteriorly, joined by the intervertebral disks as bricks are joined by mortar, with the bony arches behind. These bony arches have paired pedicles which enclose the intervertebral foramina on each side just behind the vertebral bodies. Farther back on each side one encounters the transverse processes, and finally in the mid-line of the back, the spinous processes. The whole column is bound together with various ligaments of great strength, on the anterior and posterior surfaces of the vertebral bodies and on the bony arches, their processes, and their joints. The muscles further strengthen and cushion the vertebral column.

Within the vertebral column, the circles formed by the bony arches described above are aligned to constitute a canal, called the spinal canal. The spinal canal contains the spinal cord, the trunk of nerves which is in continuity with the brain above. Neither the brain nor the spinal cord are in contact with the bones which protect them. These delicate nerve structures are completely enveloped by three concentric membranes, the meninges; respectively, the dura mater, the arachnoid, and the pia mater.

The dura mater is the most exterior membrane. Except over the first two cervical vertebrae, it is not attached to the walls of the spinal canal, but is separated from them by a space filled with fluid fat. Small fibrous bands fix it to the ligaments anteriorly. As each nerve trunk leaves the spinal cord, it receives a sheath of dura mater, a fibrous sleeve which accompanies it as far as the exit of the intervertebral foramen and there attaches to the periosteum.

The second meningeal layer, the arachnoid, adheres to the inner surface of the dura mater, separated from it only by a film of serous liquid. Further within, adherent to the spinal cord and to the nerves extending from it, is the third meningeal membrane, the pia mater. There is an appreciable space between the pia and the arachnoid, and it is in this space that the cerebrospinal fluid flows. The pia mater is connected to the dura mater by bands which cross the arachnoid.

At the exit of the intervertebral foramen, all of these membranes terminate on the nerve trunk; the pia, however, is continuous with the neurilemma, the membrane which covers the nerves beyond the limits of that foramen. There is appreciable play between the nerve and the bony walls of the intervertebral foramen. It will be shown later that it is illogical to postulate that constrictions can be produced at this site by small displacements of the vertebrae.

Turning now to the spinal nerves which pass through the interverte-bral foramina, we find that there are 31 pairs—8 cervical (the first situated between the skull and the first cervical vertebra), 12 dorsal, 5 lumbar, 5 sacral, and 1 coccygeal. In addition, there are 12 pairs of cranial nerves which have their orifices in the base of the skull.

These 12 pairs of cranial nerves and the 5 pairs of sacral nerves are manifestly out of reach of chiropractic treatment, since the bones which form their orifices have in both cases fused into a single bone. Thus of the total of 43 pairs of nerves, only 26 pairs of spinal nerves can be influenced. It remains to be determined whether illnesses can be fostered or caused by pinching or irritation of these 26 pairs of nerves.

The spinal nerves are extensions of the spinal cord. The spinal cord is a nerve trunk connected above to the brain through a large orifice in the base of the skull called the foramen magnum; it extends from the foramen magnum down most of the length of the spinal canal. The spinal cord is therefore, anatomically, a prolongation of the brain, but its function is far less complex.

The spinal nerve which passes through the intervertebral foramen is formed of two nerve roots which derive from the spinal cord and unite into a single trunk before entering the intervertebral foramen. These two roots, one anterior and one posterior, are attached to the anterior and posterior surfaces, respectively, of the spinal cord, a little to the side of the mid-line. The nerve fibers of the posterior root are sensory: they bring impulses deriving from the stimulation of end-organs of general sensation to the spinal cord and brain centers. The fibers of the anterior roots are motor; they bring impulses deriving from the stimulation of motor cells to the striated or voluntary muscles. This stimulation may be the result of a simple automatic reflex, or a complex reflex mechanism, or a voluntary act brought about by a highly organized function of the brain.

In addition to these voluntary motor fibers, the anterior roots from the first dorsal to the second lumbar segments inclusive contain other nerve fibers which are called autonomic. The autonomic fibers innervate the smooth or involuntary muscles, i.e., those of the blood vessels, digestive tract, respiratory system, urinary and genital systems, and also secretory glands. They also innervate the heart. The result of their stimulation may be either an activation or an inhibition of the function concerned.

It must also be noted that these autonomic fibers which arise from the thoraco-lumbar region of the spinal cord distribute themselves widely throughout the body, thus forming the peripheral elements of that part of the autonomic system which is called sympathetic. But these are not the only autonomic fibers which innervate the smooth muscles and the glands. A separate system of autonomic fibers, called parasympathetic, are contained in the third, seventh, ninth, and tenth pairs of cranial nerves and in the second, third, and fourth pairs of sacral nerves. As we have seen, these nerves have their orifices in fused and immovable bones, and are therefore inaccessible to chiropractic. The entire parasympathetic system is thus beyond the influence of subluxations and of chiropractic.

According to chiropractic theory, a major cause of illness is the structural disturbance of that part of the vertebral column which is accessible to manipulation, and this disturbance provokes an alteration of nervous flow in the body in different ways. The brain and the spinal cord are nerve centers which innervate the body through 43 pairs of nerve trunks. Of these, only 26 pairs of spinal nerves can be the objects of chiropractic theory, which is therefore remarkably limited in scope. The brain, the spinal cord, 12 pairs of cranial nerves, and 5 pairs of sacral nerves are anatomically protected from subluxations and from chiropractic manipulation. But these inaccessible structures are of very great importance.

The importance of the brain and spinal cord is self-evident. The cranial nerves not only innervate the head, including the senses of smell, taste, hearing, and sight; but the tenth pair of cranial nerves, the vagus nerves, innervate also the organs of the neck, the respiratory apparatus, the heart and other structures of the thorax, and a large number of abdominal organs such as the stomach, the small intestine, part of the large intestine, the pancreas, the gallbladder, the liver, the spleen, and the kidneys. The sacral nerves innervate the pelvic organs and a considerable part of the lower limbs.

These details are set forth, not for the pleasure of confounding the chiropractors, but to set straight the record of anatomic truth. Why should the 26 pairs of spinal nerves accessible to manipulation have so much importance, and the rest so little? But the fundamental question must now be studied: can subluxation cause disease?

According to chiropractic theory, as outlined before, "structural defects" impair the distribution of nervous impulses. In other words, imbalances or displacements of vertebrae diminish or accentuate nervous impulses or their effects.

Let us first examine the former situation, that of diminution. In this case there may be in the intervertebral foramen (or elsewhere, for that matter) a partial or total blockage of nervous impulses. If there is partial blockage of impulses in a nerve fiber, the research of many neurophysiologists (Verworm, Kato, Fredericq, and numerous other eminent scientists of various countries) showed several decades ago that the impulse is transmitted more slowly in a zone of partial blockage, and resumes all its characteristics as soon as it reaches normal tissue. This is comparable to the effect of a damp zone in a powder train; the combustion would be slowed by the dampness, but would flare up in full force again as soon as it reached dry powder.

Thus, it is impossible for a partial blockage of nerve impulses in a particular zone of the nerve to affect the flow, since the impulses would resume their normal flow beyond the affected zone. The slowing effect would be limited to a distance of a few millimeters in the canal of the intervertebral foramen.

There remains the case of total obstruction of nervous flow. When no impulses pass in a nerve fiber, certain specific effects occur. The muscle it innervates becomes immediately paralyzed and limp, loses its reflex responses, and soon diminishes in thickness. Sensations are also lost. Trophic disturbances may also be observed: the skin becomes dry, thin, and abnormally smooth; the nails develop longitudinal ridges and become curved and brittle. The secretion of sweat is also disturbed.

These general effects, and others as well, according to the particular function of the affected nerve, may be observed daily in our hospitals—not only as acute cases, but also as chronic cases in which the nerve pathways had been interrupted a long time before. A nerve which has been cut may be sewn together again, and the regeneration and return to function of the fibers may be observed. Never has any cause-and-effect relationship between loss of nerve function and other diseases been established. Only the specific disturbance caused by the particular loss of innervation can be demonstrated.

Obstruction in the intervertebral foramen with blockage of nerve impulses used to be the only basic hypothesis of chiropractic theory. More recently, however, chiropractors have tended to postulate a state of excitation in the intervertebral foramen. This state of excitation has never been proven by direct observation, nor has it been reproduced experimentally by proponents of chiropractic. What, then, is this other hypothesis worth?

Excitation of motor fibers produces contraction or tension in the muscle; excitation of sensory fibers sends sensory messages to the spinal cord via the posterior nerve roots. These sensory stimuli may cause a reflex response (that is to say, a direct stimulation of the corresponding motor fiber to the muscle or organ), or may be relayed to the brain, where they would give rise to various sensations, notably that of pain.

Finally, there are the sympathetic nerves of the dorso-lumbar region which have been described above; they supply the vessels and the organs. The effects of their stimulation and of their interruption have been most thoroughly and successfully studied, beginning with the work of Claude Bernard in the earliest days of modern physiology. The resultant illnesses are clear-cut, few in number, and well documented. They are, in fact, rather rare.

In addition, scientific studies have shown some years ago that the action of these nerves is communicated to the vessels and organs by the intermediary of noradrenalin, a substance liberated at the nerve endings when the nerves are stimulated, or by acetylcholine in the case of the adrenal medulla. Scientists have also isolated or synthesized a whole series of drugs which block or neutralize the action of noradrenalin or of acetylcholine, and which are administered to patients when specifically required.

There is, therefore, nothing whatsoever in the scientific facts established by the masters of normal and abnormal neurophysiology—facts which can be consistently reproduced experimentally, or observed clinically in patients—to sustain chiropractic's fundamental hypothesis that obstructions in the mechanical structure of the human body are true causes of disease.

Indeed, in the field of human biology, chiropractic theory ignores a host of other facts discovered by human intelligence, facts which have infinitely widened the horizons of our knowledge and have provided explanations for many of nature's most important phenomena.

In biology there are, in addition to the nervous system, other systems, perhaps even more fundamental, which are relatively independent of the nervous system and which regulate bodily function. The research of the last three-quarters of a century has demonstrated the existence and the methods of function of the whole system of regulation of biologic activities by the endocrine glands. The materials secreted by these glands (hormones) enter directly into the circulation and are absorbed by the appropriate organs, and regulate the function of those organs by direct action on their cells.

These effects do not require the participation of the nervous system. In numerous experiments, they have been observed in tissues removed from the body and separated from all connections with the nervous system. Hundreds of thousands of studies have been done on the endocrine glands and their hormones; no scientist has ever traced a disease of (or related to) the endocrine glands to a mechanical obstruction affecting a peripheral nerve trunk.

Still more basic than these two regulatory systems, nervous and endocrine, is the inherent automatism which governs the function of organs as important as the heart, the digestive system, the urinary system, the smooth muscles, and the blood vessels. For example, the perfused heart, even though cut off from all nervous or endocrine influence and even if removed from the body, continues to beat as long as it is surrounded by a suitable medium. This was shown in the classic perfusion experiments. The same phenomena may be obtained with the other organs mentioned.

This is not to minimize the importance of the nervous system, nor of the system of endocrine glands. But their importance does not vitiate that of these other mechanisms, which may be considered more fundamental and are much more stable.

At the cellular level, to which chiropractic theory claims to extend, the same conclusions must be drawn. The media of public information have made the average citizen aware of the existence of the electron microscope and of the possibilities of its use in the study of cellular biology. In the body of a cell there are a whole series of submicroscopic components: mitochondria, microsomes, lysosomes, particles of endoplasmic reticulum, etc. Chemists have succeeded in isolating them and subjecting them to analysis. These particles contain enzymes, biochemical catalysts of reactions within the cell.

Nowhere in these extraordinary studies, constituting as they did an objective and systematic search for truth, was chiropractic theory validated. On the contrary, it was possible to attribute certain diseases to absences of certain enzymes from body cells. This type of cellular research has reached so high a degree of precision that it has been possible to specify which chemical molecule is responsible for a particular disease. Thus it has been found that the cause of certain blood diseases resides in the chemical composition of the hemoglobin molecule of the red cell—more specifically in the absence of one of the amino acids which are component fragments of the hemoglobin molecule.

Not all illnesses are as yet so precisely understood, but one can already envisage the day when their causes will be understood down to the molecular level. These intracellular mechanisms are fundamental, and are completely independent of the nervous system. Chiropractic, therefore, scrutinized in relation to the cell itself, remains a contradiction to science.

Even though it is in opposition to true science, could not chiropractic have a practical value comparable to that of scientifically-oriented medicine?

Chiropractic in Relation to Clinical Science
Every day physicians see patients suffering from disorders of the nervous system, including those of the peripheral nerves. They have available to them all known physical and chemical methods of investigation, including the recording of nerve impulses in the brain, peripheral nerves, and muscles. Tissues removed at operation and at autopsy are carefully and compulsorily examined by a pathologist, who studies their cellular conditions and correlates his diagnosis with clinical observations and operative findings.

There are indeed cases of obstruction to nerve flow, and of irritations of surrounding tissues. But these result in specific disturbances—paralysis, muscle wasting, pain, sensory disturbances, vascular disorders, etc.—but no diseases other than these which are directly related to the function of the nerve in question. Fortunately, these patients are not afflicted with all the ills known to man. The nervous system is important; it has a specific role to play; but it is far from being the sole system of control. To illustrate this truth, a paraplegic woman (whose spinal cord has been interrupted and is deprived of any effect of higher nerve centers) may conceive, carry her pregnancy to term, and give birth to a normal baby.

Orthopedists, whose field is to examine and operate on the vertebral column, frequently encounter the whole range of diseases from benign and superficial inflammation of tissues to malignancies of those bones—including particularly herniation of the intervertebral disk, a condition which should logically produce obstructions. The vertebral column is treated, and the obstruction, if there is one, relieved. But if other troubles exist, they do not disappear merely with the correction of the vertebral column.

To go further, the causes of a very large number of illnesses are now well known. An immense army of scholars—physicians, chemists, physicists, biologists mathematicians, indeed men of every scientific discipline—contribute to this knowledge throughout the world. Their work is subjected to a meticulousness of thought which tries to leave nothing to chance. The causes they have found have been widely varied trauma, poisons, nutritional deficiencies, bacteria, viruses, congenital defects, etc. In each case strict proof has been established between the cause or causes and the disease manifestations. Never has chiropractic theory found a place here. With the greatest indulgence in the world, no place can be found for chiropractic in the practical treatment of disease.

It should certainly not be concluded that medicine ignores or rejects vertebral therapy; but this treatment is far removed from chiropractic, both in principle and in application. Mechanical treatment of vertebrae, whether by manipulation or by traction, is only one of many methods used by physical medicine, which is itself only a small part of the therapeutic armamentarium available to the physician for the treatment of painful conditions of vertebral origin.

The vertebral column, because of its particular structure (numerous articulations, disks which tend to degenerate, etc.), its role as a structural support, and the enormous strains and pressures to which it is subjected, is frequently the seat of pain. The regions most susceptible are the neck and the lumbo-sacral axis.

Certain of these painful conditions may be relieved and sometimes cured by maneuvering the affected region. These forcible passive movements are called manipulations. Manipulation as a therapeutic technique is effective in some cases, but most often is a single element in a program of treatment aimed at restoring the spine to both static and dynamic normalcy. In medicine, these treatments must be decided upon and carried out by a physician; they are never given over to a technician.

The pattern of treatment varies with the clinical problem. Nevertheless, certain general rules should be observed. The first is that the proper use of manipulation depends on accurate diagnosis. Every case of vertebral pain requires a careful history, physical examination and x-rays, and such laboratory tests as may be necessary. It should be borne in mind that:

(a) Each pain of vertebral origin, whether local, distributed along the nerve, or referred elsewhere, is not necessarily dependent on a type of spinal involvement susceptible to manipulation. In consequence, a precise diagnosis must be made before it can be decided whether treatment by manipulation is justified.

(b) Any inflammation, tumor, or infectious lesion of the spine may first show itself by virtue of a strain or unusual movement. In such cases, it would be dangerous to fail to recognize the true diagnosis.

(c) Treatment by manipulation is not an irreplaceable form of therapy. It is certainly tempting because its effects may be rapid and sometimes even immediate. It should be done only if it can be well done. It is better to use other methods than to manipulate badly: "*Primum non nocere.*"

Only if all precautions have been taken should treatment by manipulation be decided on.

Thus, proper manipulation, which aims at relieving pain and improving function, requires sound understanding of the condition for which manipulation is to be done. This also implies complete familiarity with the anatomy and the mechanics of the vertebral column.

Manipulation of the vertebral column may be indicated: (a) in localized stiffness of the spine, with accompanying pain; (b) in disturbances associated with the protrusion of a disk; and (3) in sprains of the spine, i.e., traumatic or static conditions in which the disk does not appear to be involved.

These Are the Only Three Indications
It is important to repeat here that no form of treatment is irreplaceable. There are certainly cases which can be cured or relieved by manipulation. Very often, however, other treatments can achieve the same result. It is better to refrain from manipulation than to do harm by it, and indications for manipulation must be based on an exact medical diagnosis.

In painful conditions of the vertebral column, traction is also a widely-used form of therapy in medicine. The three principal indications for traction are: (a) to put the spine at rest by immobilization, (b) to overcome muscle spasm, and (c) to use sufficient pull to separate bony surfaces. Thus, mechanical therapy of the vertebral column, either as manipulation or as traction, may be indicated in certain painful conditions of vertebral origin.

It must again be emphasized that in medicine, treatment of the vertebral column is not used to deal with conditions situated elsewhere. Medicine treats disease in terms of its cause.

The Achievements and Uses of Chiropractic
Every worthwhile scientific achievement, no matter how small, pushes back the boundaries of our ignorance, extends the horizon of our knowledge, and puts known facts into new perspectives which lead to further experimental studies. As research budgets climb in geometric progression, limited only by the economic possibilities of each country, we are witnessing an explosion of discoveries which evokes in contemporary man a wondering admiration.

Since the beginning of this century, man has acquired more understanding of nature than he had previously achieved since the Creation. A mere listing of new concepts in human biology added in this century to our store of knowledge would be overwhelming. It is common knowledge that many diseases have been entirely conquered, that others are gradually disappearing, and that surgery in recent years has shown prodigious achievements. It is hard to think of a single area in which progress has not been made. These facts are too well known to bear further elaboration.

Chiropractic was invented in the early days of this scientific revolution. It professes interest in the nervous system, bones, joints, and muscles. Yet it is impossible to cite a single worthwhile scientific discovery, a single contribution by chiropractic to our understanding of the mechanics and functions of these organs. When allusion is made to the progress of chiropractic, it is in terms of increases in the numbers of chiropractors, of patients, and of states which have legalized chiropractic. Never has a chiropractor requested a research grant from the National Research Council of Canada, nor from that of the United States. Even today, chiropractors offer no prospect of contributing to science, as witness their Bill 216.

Practically speaking, what can chiropractic offer a patient? A person appears who may be suffering from a variety of illnesses, some benign and tending towards spontaneous cure, others grave and even mortal. For all of these diseases, since 1895, chiropractic has offered a single treatment—the manipulation of 24 vertebrae. It is the claim of chiropractic that health in human society can be protected simply by maintaining the alignment of these 24 vertebrae.

Summary

In the course of this brief, the College of Physicians and Surgeons of the Province of Quebec has set forth its views on the question of chiropractic.

The scientific value of chiropractic has been examined at the outset. Defined in Bill 216, presented in February 1963 to the Quebec legislature, as "the art of detecting and localizing obstructions which, in the mechanical structure of the human body, alter the distribution and normal physiologic action of nervous inflow to tissues and cells; of correcting these obstructions by manipulation, particularly in the region of the vertebral column; and of advising the measures necessary to prevent their return; the whole without the aid of medications nor of surgery," chiropractic rests on four postulates:

(1) Displacements or subluxations of the vertebrae disturb the distribution of nervous flow;

(2) Disturbances of the distribution of nerve flow impair health and cause disease;

(3) Chiropractic technique detects, localizes, and permanently reduces these subluxations;

(4) Chiropractic treatment re-establishes the normal distribution of nervous flow and restores the health.

None of these interdependent postulates is supported by scientific proof. To go even further, scientific evidence, both experimental and clinical, is wholly opposed to the theory in principle and in application. Because of its essential fallacy, chiropractic has contributed nothing to the progress of science. The College of Physicians and Surgeons of the Province of Quebec, therefore, cannot accept chiropractic as a valid method for the treatment of patients.

The College of Physicians and Surgeons submits also that the education of chiropractors is unacceptable because in schools of chiropractic the numbers and training of the teachers, as well as the organization of the courses, are far below minimum standards.

It has also been demonstrated in this brief that chiropractic is dangerous, because it leaves the patient without a diagnosis and without the treatment specifically indicated for his or her particular illness, and because the maneuvers of which it consists are themselves potentially dangerous. A clear distinction has been made between vertebral manipulation as a medical procedure, used in well-defined conditions and in appropriate cases, and vertebral manipulation as a chiropractic cure-all with its basis in false hypotheses.

Lastly, the peculiarities of legislation concerning chiropractic have been discussed. The wide variations in privileges granted to, and restrictions imposed on, chiropractic in the states and provinces in which it has been legalized shows that legislatures have more or less tolerated chiropractors but have not endorsed chiropractic. This conclusion is reinforced by the fact that in the wars of 1914–18 and 1939–45 no chiropractor was employed as such in the Canadian and American armed forces.

The lack of financial support to schools of chiropractic by state and provincial governments also confirms the impression. No university, no scientific group nor society supports chiropractic theory.

Some consequences of the legal recognition of chiropractic in this province have been set forth. The College of Physicians and Surgeons of the Province of Quebec rejects chiropractic because: (1) chiropractic is a false theory; (2) the education of chiropractors is below acceptable standards; and (3) chiropractic is potentially dangerous.

The College can accept no part of the responsibility for legal recognition of chiropractic in the Province of Quebec, neither before the people of the province nor before the tribunal of history.

Appendix B

A Scientific Test of Chiropractic's Subluxation Theory

The first experimental study of the basis of the theory demonstrates that it is erroneous.

Edmund S. Crelin, Ph.D.

Chiropractic is defined in the dictionary as "a therapeutic system based upon the premise that disease is caused by the interference with nerve function, the method being to restore normal condition by adjusting the segments of the spinal column" [1]. The International Chiropractors Association defines chiropractic as follows:

> The philosophy of chiropractic is based upon the premise that disease or abnormal function is caused by interference with nerve transmission and expression, due to pressure, strain or tension upon the spinal cord or spinal nerves, as a result of body segments of the vertebral column deviating from their normal juxtaposition. The practice of chiropractic consists of analysis of an interference with normal nerve transmission and expression, and the correction thereof by an adjustment with the hands of the abnormal deviations of the bony articulations of the vertebral column for the restoration and maintenance of health, without the use of drugs or surgery. The term "analysis" is construed to include the use of X-ray and other analytical instruments generally used in the practice of chiropractic. [2,3,7]

The definition given by the American Chiropractic Association is:

> Chiropractic practice is the specific adjustment and manipulation of the articulations and adjacent tissues of the body, particularly of

the spinal column, for the correction of nerve interference and includes the use of recognized diagnostic methods, as indicated. Patient care is conducted with due regard for environmental, nutritional, and psychotherapeutic factors, as well as first aid, hygiene, sanitation, rehabilitation and related procedures designed to restore or maintain normal nerve function. [2,4,7]

According to chiropractic, the deviation of the body segments of the vertebral column from their normal juxtaposition that interferes with nerve transmission and expression is called subluxation. Two chiropractic descriptions of subluxation are:

"The vertebrae are . . . within their normal range of motion, although not functioning at their optimum." [5]

"A vertebral subluxation may be interpreted as 'off-centering of a vertebral segment.' [A subluxation] is a fixation of the joint within its normal range of movement, usually at the extremity of this range." [6]

In other words, subluxed vertebrae (spinal bones) are characterized by fixation and misalignment within the normal range of motion.

Daniel David Palmer, a tradesman who posed as a magnetic healer, "discovered" chiropractic in 1895. Magnetic healing was a popular form of quackery in the nineteenth century in which the healers believed that their personal magnetism was so great that it gave them the power to cure disease [7]. Palmer said:

I am the originator, the Fountain Head of the essential principle that disease is the result of too much or not enough functionating [sic]. I created the art of adjusting vertebrae, using the spinous and transverse processes as levers, and named the mental act of accumulating knowledge, the cumulative function, corresponding to the physical vegetative function—growth of intellectual and physical-together, with the science, art and philosophy—Chiropractic. . . . It was I who combined the science and art and developed the principles thereof. I have answered the question—what is life? [8]

The chiropractic philosophy originated by Palmer is the frame of reference of modern-day chiropractic thinking as exemplified in the most widely used chiropractic textbook [5] at the present time. Palmer put forth the concepts of Universal Intelligence, Innate Intelligence, and Educated Intelligence. Universal Intelligence is God. Innate Intelligence is the "Soul, Spirit or Spark of Life" or "Nature, intuition, instinct, spiritual and subconscious mind." It is the "something" within the body which controls the healing process, growth, and repair and "is beyond the finite knowledge."

While Innate Intelligence utilizes the autonomic nervous system, the Educated Intelligence, or "conscious," utilizes "the cerebrospinal division for the volitional expression of its function."

Nature, or Innate Intelligence, has a great capacity to maintain or restore health if it is allowed normal expression within the body. However, mental, chemical, or mechanical stress can produce a greater or lesser displacement of the vertebrae, or vertebral disrelationship, and this displacement interferes with the planned expression of Innate Intelligence through the nerves. This interference then produces pathology. The chiropractor, by correcting the displacement, allows the Innate Intelligence to effect the cure [5,9]. The pathology that chiropractors treat by manual manipulation of the spine totals over ninety diseases, including gastrointestinal, genitourinary, respiratory, vascular, and emotional disorders; diabetes; deafness; eye disorders; cancer; arthritis; and infectious diseases such as polio, mumps, hepatitis, diphtheria, and the common cold [7,10].

No one, and this includes chiropractors, has ever experimentally determined how much vertebral displacement is necessary before a spinal nerve is impinged or encroached upon at the intervertebral foramen to produce pathology by interfering with the planned expression of Innate Intelligence. This study was performed to answer that question.

Of the 43 pairs of nerves that pass from the brain and spinal cord to the various parts of the body, only 24 pairs could ever be impinged or encroached upon by the displacement of one vertebra against another as the nerves pass out of the intervertebral foramina. There is a superior and an inferior articular process posterolaterally on each side of a vertebra. Anterior to each articular process there is a notch; therefore, when the processes articulate with those of adjacent vertebrae above and below to form the vertebral column, a series of holes is formed—the intervertebral foramina. [Note: "Foramen" is the medical term for an opening through a bony structure or membrane. The plural is foramina. The intervertebral foramina are the openings between the spinal bones through which the spinal nerves emerge from the spinal cord to connect to other parts of the body.]

Part of the anterior margin of an intervertebral foramen is formed by the intervertebral disk that joins the two bodies of adjacent vertebrae together. In addition to the way the bony parts articulate with one another, numerous ligaments and muscles, both long and short, serve to bind adjacent vertebrae together to restrict their movement. Although the displacement between adjacent vertebrae is small, the range of total motion of the entire vertebral column is considerable.

Throughout life the intervertebral foramina are quite large in relationship to the spinal nerves that pass through them [11]. . . . A tiny artery and an intervertebral vein usually accompany each spinal nerve through the foramen. The remainder of the space of each foramen contains very flimsy, loose areolar tissue.

Materials and Methods

The vertebral columns of six individuals were studied. Three were infants, one a full-term newborn female who failed to breathe after birth; the other two, a male and a female, were full-term infants who died of a respiratory disorder within a week after birth. The remainder were adults: a 35-year-old male who died following a heart attack, a 73-year-old male who died of pneumonitis, and a 76-year-old female who died of infectious hepatitis. The vertebral column of each individual was excised within 3 to 6 hours after death. Shortly after death each cadaver was cooled to 40°F until the vertebral column was excised.

From a posterior approach the first cervical vertebra was disarticulated from the skull, and the fifth lumbar vertebra was disarticulated from the sacrum. Each spinal nerve was transected at a point 8 cm after it emerged from its intervertebral foramen. The ribs were also transected, leaving 5 cm of their proximal ends attached to the vertebral column. All of the deep musculature of the vertebral column was left intact except the bulk of the psoas major muscles and the caudal part of the erector spinae muscles. None of the ligaments and joint capsules of the vertebral column was disturbed. Therefore, the test of the displacement of individual vertebrae in this experiment was actually a test of the passive action of the attached ligaments to limit any displacement. In a living individual there would have been the added resistance of the attached muscles contracting in a reflex manner to inhibit vertebral displacement, or subluxation.

As soon as the vertebral column was excised it was immersed in a physiological saline solution at body temperature to insure maximum flexibility of its joints during the testing that immediately followed. A careful inspection both before and after the testing revealed that each vertebral column was normal for the age of the individual from which it was excised.

A standard drill press was used for the tests. It had a rotating handle that allowed the forceful lowering of the chuck, to which was attached a Dillon force gauge certified to be accurate to within ±1% of full scale reading. It was a compression model with marked dial increments of 10 pounds up to a capacity of 1,000 pounds. The two pressure feet used were solid metal rods that could be screwed onto the bottom of the force gauge. The end of one of the rods that exerted pressure on the vertebral column was tapered and flat; the other was forked.

The drill press had a handle that allowed the pressure foot to be locked in position while exerting continuous compression on individual vertebrae of the column. Two metal vises were clamped to the platform of the drill press to support the vertebral column while it was subjected to a compressive force. The column was only lightly clamped by the two vises supporting it. This allowed five vertebral segments of the newborn column and three of the adult column, suspended between the vises, to move freely when force was applied. The pressure foot with a forked end was used to apply compression on both sides of each vertebra by fitting it over the transverse process; it was also used to apply compression to the back of each vertebra by fitting the forked end over the spinous process. The pressure foot with the tapered flat end was used to apply compression to the front of each vertebra of a newborn column. However, a flat piece of metal the same width as each vertebral body of the adult column had to be interposed between the pressure foot and the body because almost as soon as force was applied the tapered end began to break the bone and pass into the body.

When the part of the vertebra to which the pressure foot was applied began to break or collapse, the force was stopped. After a couple of transverse or spinous processes broke early in the testing, I learned to determine by sight, sound, and feel just about the time it was going to happen again. Each vertebral body was quite compressible: it could be compressed to about two-thirds its anteroposterior width and still rebound to its original width when the pressure was released. If compressed beyond this point, it would remain in a collapsed condition.

A Dresser torque wrench was used to quantify the amount of torsional force applied when the vertebral column was twisted. The wrench face was marked in increments of 5 foot-pounds up to 140 pounds and certified to be accurate within ±1%. The adult column was held snugly in a vise with its anterior surface facing upward. The transverse processes were hooked under the jaws of the vise to prevent the column from turning when torsional force was applied to the portion of the column projecting beyond the vise. A chain clamp was firmly applied to each vertebra in turn, beginning with the first cervical and ending with the fifth lumbar. The chain clamp had a fitting into which the end of the torque wrench was inserted. A twisting force was applied both to the right and left. The maximum force applied was at the point when it was obvious that the tissues of the column were about to rupture. While the maximal torsional force was being exerted, the spinal nerves and their intervertebral foramina were observed. The entire newborn column was easily twisted manually both to the right and left and then held in the extreme position by clamping each end of the column in a vise while the spinal nerves and intervertebral foramina were observed.

An Ametek push-pull gauge was used to quantify the amount of force applied when the vertebral column was bent in all directions. The dial was marked in 2-pound increments up to 200 pounds and certified to be accurate to within ± 0.5% of full scale. The adult column was held in a vise in the same manner as it was for the application of a torsional force. The portion of the column projecting beyond the vise was attached to the push-pull gauge by a cord wrapped around it. Segments of the column were made to project beyond the vise and maximally flexed, extended, and laterally bent both left and right to the point that the tissues of the column were about to rupture. While the segment of the column was maximally bent in one direction, the spinal nerves and their intervertebral foramina were observed. As shown in the picture below, the newborn column was so flexible that it could easily be bent in a half-circle in flexion, extension, and left and right

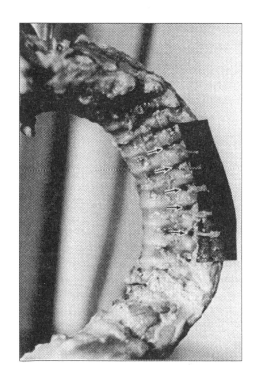

When 30 to 40 pounds of pressure were applied by the drill press foot to the cervical end of the newborn columns, they became maximally curved in flexion, extension, and lateral bending to form a half-circle. No reduction in the size of the intervertebral foramina in maximum flexion and extension was significant, because there was always a relatively large space surrounding the nerves in the foramina.

The cervical end is at the top. A black piece of paper was placed behind the 5th to 9th left thoracic spinal nerves where they emerge from their intervertebral foramina to make them more visible.

laterally [11]. It could be held in any position of maximal bending by placing it between the pressure foot and the platform of the drill press while the spinal nerves and their intervertebral foramina were observed.

A Mura volt-ohm-microampere meter was used when the first vertebral column, from the 35-year-old male adult, was tested. The meter was used to determine whether the border of the intervertebral foramen came into contact with the spinal nerve when compressive, bending, or twisting forces were applied to the vertebral column. The wire from the positive pole of the meter was wrapped around the spinal nerve that was placed against one side of the intervertebral foramen; the wire from the negative pole of the meter was placed against the opposite side of the foramen. The meter was set at 1,000 ohms, and if the wires barely touched each other the recording needle would make a full swing across the face of the dial. The tests of the first vertebral column revealed that the relationship of a spinal nerve to the borders of its intervertebral foramen could very easily be determined with the naked eye at all times during the continuous application of force. Therefore it was not necessary to use the meter when testing the other columns.

All the spinal nerves emerging from their intervertebral foramina were exposed prior to the testing of each vertebral column. Gentle teasing with a pair of small forceps easily removed the flimsy areolar tissue surrounding the nerves to expose the borders of their relatively spacious intervertebral foramina. At any time during the testing when a constant force of compression, twisting, or bending was being applied to the column, the very soft and extremely flexible spinal nerves could easily be moved about. The cut ends of the nerves were grasped with forceps and held in all positions to determine by direct observation any encroachment or impingement smaller foramina might have on the nerves.

Findings

The range of maximum compressive force, or breaking point, that could be applied to the individual vertebrae of the cervical, thoracic, and lumbar regions of the newborn and adult columns before they became irreversibly collapsed is shown in the table on page 204. While a continuous maximum force was applied to a vertebra by locking the drill press handle in position, the adjacent spinal nerves and their intervertebral foramina were examined and measured. There was a slight lateral displacement of an individual vertebra when maximum pressure was applied to one of its transverse

Range of Maximum Compressive Force
Before Breaking Point of Individual Vertebrae

Site of force	Pounds of compressive force	
	Newborn	Adult
Vertebral bodies		
Cervical	30–50	100–115
Thoracic	30–50	130–300
Lumbar	30–50	210–295
Transverse processes		
Cervical	20–25	98–125
Thoracic	20–25	100–185
Lumbar	20–25	148–185
Spinous processes		
Cervical	15–20	100–115
Thoracic	15–20	95–110
Lumbar	15–20	100–150

processes, along with a slight increase in the size of the adjacent intervertebral foramen in relationship to its nerve.

There was slight displacement of an individual vertebra that resulted in a reduction in the size of the adjacent foramina when the highly unphysiologic maximum pressure was applied to its body or spinous process. However, the nerves passing through these foramina could be freely moved about while the force was being continuously applied, because in the adult columns the foramina were quite spacious in relation to their spinal nerves. There was never less than 1.5 mm of space completely surrounding the cervical nerves, 3 mm of space surrounding the thoracic nerves, and 4 mm surrounding the lumbar nerves. In the newborn columns there was also a relatively large amount of space surrounding the spinal nerves during the application of a maximum compressive force. There was never less than 1 mm of space surrounding the cervical nerves and 2 mm clearance surrounding the thoracic and lumbar nerves. Upon release of the compressive force the vertebrae of both the adult and newborn columns immediately returned to their original position, and the adjacent foramina immediately returned to their original size.

The greatest amount of twisting motion of the entire adult vertebral column occurred in the upper cervical region at a maximum torsional force of 35 to 45 pounds. The next greatest amount was in the upper lumbar region, and the least in the thoracic region. When the maximal torsional force of about 10 pounds was applied to the newborn columns, the degree of twisting motion was the same throughout their length and was comparatively much greater than that of the adult column, especially in the thoracic region.

Any reduction in the size of the intervertebral foramina during the application of torsional force to both the adult and newborn columns was insignificant in relation to the spinal nerves passing through the foramina. There was always a relatively large amount of space surrounding the nerves in the foramina. As the torsional force was gradually applied, careful observation revealed that the amount of sliding motion of the nerves was insignificant in relation to the foramina. My observations indicated that the nerves did not become unduly stretched when the column was maximally twisted.

The greatest amount of flexion of the adult columns occurred in the lower cervical and the mid-lumbar regions when a maximal bending force of 50 to 60 pounds was applied. There was only moderate flexion in the thoracic region of the column from the 35-year-old male and even less in the thoracic region of the columns from the two older individuals. The greatest extension of the adult columns was seen in the cervical region, with the next greatest in the lumbar region when a maximum bending force of 50 pounds was applied. A moderate extension occurred in the thoracic region of the column from the 35-year-old male, whereas that in the thoracic region of the columns from the two older individuals was hardly detectable. The greatest lateral bending was in the cervical region of the adult columns, with the next greatest in the lumbar region when a maximum force of 50 to 60 pounds was applied. There was only a moderate amount in the thoracic region.

Any reduction in the size of the intervertebral foramina during the application of a bending force to produce flexion, extension, and lateral bending of the adult columns was insignificant in relation to the spinal nerves passing through the foramina. This was true also on the concave side of the lateral bend, where the greatest reduction in foramen size occurred. Under all conditions a relatively large amount of space surrounded the nerves in the foramina. The nerves were observed as the column was bent, and the sliding motion was seen to be insignificant relative to the possibility that the nerves might be unduly stretched when the column was maximally bent.

On the convex side of the laterally bent newborn column there was a significant increase in the size of the foramina, whereas on the concave side there was a significant decrease, to the point that the borders of the foramina made contact with nerves passing through them. However, the nerves were not markedly impinged upon and could be made to slide back and forth within the foramina when they were grasped with forceps. The extreme degree of lateral bending needed to cause encroachment of the foramina on the nerves could not occur in an intact infant because the internal organs and the body wall with its ribs would not permit it.

This experimental study demonstrates conclusively that the subluxation of a vertebra as defined by chiropractic—the exertion of pressure on a spinal nerve which by interfering with the planned expression of Innate Intelligence produces pathology—does not occur. This is what should be expected when one recognizes that the vertebral column has been evolving for over 400 million years to support the body and protect the central nervous system. By a process of natural selection the vertebral column of mammals has evolved into one in which the articulations allow an overall range of motion so that individuals may function well for survival within their environment. At the same time the selective process has favored vertebral columns that have spacious intervertebral foramina in combination with the barest minimum of displacement between adjacent vertebrae-two factors that preclude impingement upon the spinal nerves as they pass through the foramina.

References

1. *The Random House Dictionary of the English Language.* 1966. New York: Random House.
2. Data Sheet on Chiropractic. 1970. Chicago: Department of Investigation, American Medical Association.
3. International Chiropractors Review. International Chiropractors Association. March 1964, p. 2.
4. Journal of the American Chiropractic Association. Nov 1963, p. 13.
5. Homewood AE. 1962. *The Neurodynamics of the Vertebral Subluxation.* Published by the author.
6. Harper WD. 1964. *Anything Can Cause Anything.* San Antonio, Texas: published by the author.
7. Smith RL. *At Your Own Risk: The Case against Chiropractic.* New York: Pocket Books, 1969.
8. Palmer DD. *The Science, Art and Philosophy of Chiropractic.* Reprint of 1910 edition. Portland, Oregon: Portland Printing House, 1966.
9. Cohen WJ. *Independent Practitioners under Medicare: A Report to Congress.* Washington, DC: Department of Health, Education, and Welfare, 1968.

10. Chiropractic Survey and Statistical Study. 1963. A report to the Board of Directors, National Chiropractic Association. (Mimeographed) Des Moines: Bratten and Associates, 1963, pp. 32–35.
11. Crelin ES 1973. *Functional Anatomy of the Newborn.* New Haven, Conn.: Yale University Press, 1973.
12. Crelin ES. *Anatomy of the Newborn: An Atlas.* Philadelphia: Lea and Febiger, 1969.

This article was published with additional illustrations in the September/October 1973 issue of *American Scientist*, the journal of the Society of Sigma Xi. At that time, Dr. Crelin was Professor of Anatomy and Chairman of the Human Growth and Development Study Unit at the Yale University School of Medicine. He had published over 100 papers on the development, structure, and physiology of bones and joints and was the author of the first atlas of the anatomy of the human newborn ever published.

Appendix C

AHCPR Guidelines
for Low Back Pain

From:

Acute Low Back Problems in Adults
Clinical Practice Guideline
Quick Reference Guide Number 14
AHCPR Publication No. 95-0643, December 1994

U.S. Department of Health and Human Services
Public Health Service
Agency for Health Care Policy and Research
Rockville, Maryland

Purpose and Scope

Low back problems affect virtually everyone at some time during their life. Surveys indicate a yearly prevalence of symptoms in 50 percent of working age adults; 15-20 percent seek medical care. Low back problems rank high among the reasons for physician office visits and are costly in terms of medical treatment, lost productivity, and nonmonetary costs such as diminished ability to perform or enjoy usual activities. In fact, for persons under age 45, low back problems are the most common cause of disability.

Acute low back problems are defined as activity intolerance due to lower back or back-related leg symptoms of less than 3 months' duration. About 90 percent of patients with acute low back problems spontaneously recover activity tolerance within 1 month. The approach to a new episode in a patient with a recurrent low back problem is similar to that of a new acute episode.

The findings and recommendations included in the *Clinical Practice Guideline* define a paradigm shift away from focusing care exclusively on the pain and toward helping patients improve activity tolerance. The intent of this *Quick Reference Guide* is to bring to life this paradigm shift. The guide provides information on the detection of serious conditions that occasionally cause low back symptoms (conditions such as spinal fracture, tumor, infection, cauda equina syndrome, or non-spinal conditions). However, treatment of these conditions is beyond the scope of this guideline. In addition, the guideline does not address the care of patients younger than 18 years or those with chronic back problems (back-related activity limitations of greater than 3 months' duration).

Initial Assessment

■ Seek potentially dangerous underlying conditions.

■ In the absence of signs of dangerous conditions, there is no need for special studies since 90 percent of patients will recover spontaneously within 4 weeks.

A focused medical history and physical examination are sufficient to assess the patient with an acute or recurrent limitation due to low back symptoms of less than 4 weeks duration. Patient responses and findings on the history and physical examination, referred to as "red flags" (Table 1), raise suspicion of serious underlying spinal conditions. Their absence rules out the need for special studies during the first 4 weeks of symptoms when spontaneous recovery is expected. The medical history and physical examination can also alert the clinician to non-spinal pathology (abdominal, pelvic, thoracic) that can present as low back symptoms. Acute low back symptoms can then be classified into one of three working categories:

■ *Potentially serious spinal condition*—tumor, infection, spinal fracture, or a major neurologic compromise, such as cauda equina syndrome, suggested by a red flag.

■ *Sciatica*—back-related lower limb symptoms suggesting lumbosacral nerve root compromise.

■ *Nonspecific back symptoms*—occurring primarily in the back and suggesting neither nerve root compromise nor a serious underlying condition.

Table 1. Red flags for potentially serious conditions

Possible fracture	Possible tumor or infection	Possible cauda equina syndrome
From medical history		
Major trauma, such as vehicle accident or fall from height. Minor trauma or even strenuous lifting (in older or potentially osteoporotic patient).	Age over 50 or under 20. History of cancer. Constitutional symptoms, such as recent fever or chills or unexplained weight loss. Risk factors for spinal infection: recent bacterial infection (e.g., urinary tract infection); IV drug abuse; or immune suppression (from steroids, transplant, or HIV). Pain that worsens when supine; severe nighttime pain.	Saddle anesthesia. Recent onset of bladder dysfunction, such as urinary retention, increased frequency, or overflow incontinence. Severe or progressive neurologic deficit in the lower extremity.
From physical examination		
		Unexpected laxity of the anal sphincter. Perianal/perineal sensory loss. Major motor weakness: quadriceps (knee extension weakness); ankle plantar flexors, evertors, and dorsiflexors (foot drop).

Medical History

In addition to detecting serious conditions and categorizing back symptoms, the medical history establishes rapport between the clinician and patient. The patient's description of present symptoms and limitations, duration of symptoms, and history of previous episodes defines the problem. It also provides insight into concerns, expectations, and nonphysical (psychological and socioeconomic) issues that may alter the patient's response to treatment. Assessment tools such as pain drawings and visual analog pain-rating scales may help further document the patient's perceptions and progress.

A patient's estimate of personal activity intolerance due to low back symptoms contributes to the clinical assessment of the severity of the back problem, guides treatment, and establishes a baseline for recommending daily activities and evaluating progress.

Open-ended questions, such as those listed below, can gauge the need for further discussion or specific inquiries for more detailed information:

- **What are your symptoms?**

  Pain, numbness, weakness, stiffness?

  Located primarily in back, leg, or both?

  Constant or intermittent?

- **How do these symptoms limit you?**

  How long can you sit, stand, walk?

  How much weight can you lift?

- **When did the current limitations begin?**

  How long have your activities been limited? More than 4 weeks?

  Have you had similar episodes previously?

  Previous testing or treatment?

- **What do you hope we can accomplish during this visit?**

Physical Examination

Guided by the medical history, the physical examination includes:

- General observation of the patient.
- A regional back exam.
- Neurologic screening.
- Testing for sciatic nerve root tension.

The examination is mostly subjective since patient response or interpretation is required for all parts except reflex testing and circumferential measurements for atrophy.

Addressing Red Flags

Physical examination evidence of severe neurologic compromise that correlates with the medical history may indicate a need for immediate consultation. The examination may further modify suspicions of tumor, infection, or significant trauma. A medical history suggestive of non-spinal pathology mimicking a back problem may warrant examination of pulses, abdomen, pelvis, or other areas.

Observation and Regional Back Examination

Limping or coordination problems indicate the need for specific neurologic testing. Severe guarding of lumbar motion in all planes may support a suspected diagnosis of spinal infection, tumor, or fracture. However, given marked variations among persons with and without symptoms, range-of-motion measurements of the back are of limited value.

Vertebral point tenderness to palpation, when associated with other signs or symptoms, may be suggestive of but not specific for spinal fracture or infection. Palpable soft-tissue tenderness is, by itself, an even less specific or reliable finding.

Neurologic Screening

The neurologic examination can focus on a few tests that seek evidence of nerve root impairment, peripheral neuropathy, or spinal cord dysfunction. Over 90 percent of all clinically significant lower extremity radiculopathy due to disc herniation involves the L5 or S1 nerve root at the L4-5 or L5-S1 disc

level. The clinical features of nerve root compression are summarized in Figure 1.

- ■ *Testing for Muscle Strength.* The patient's inability to toe walk (calf muscles, mostly S1 nerve root), heel walk (ankle and toe dorsiflexor muscles, L5 and some L4 nerve roots), or do a single squat and rise (quadriceps muscles, mostly L4 nerve root) may indicate muscle weakness. Specific testing of the dorsiflexor muscles of the ankle or great toe (suggestive of L5 or some L4 nerve root dysfunction), hamstrings and ankle evertors (L5-S1), and toe flexors (S1) is also important.

- ■ *Circumferential Measurements.* Muscle atrophy can be detected by circumferential measurements of the calf and thigh bilaterally. Differences of less than 2 cm in measurements of the two limbs at the same level may be a normal variation. Symmetrical muscle bulk and strength are expected unless the patient has a neurologic impairment or a history of lower extremity muscle or joint problem.

- ■ *Reflexes.* The ankle jerk reflex tests mostly the S1 nerve root and the knee jerk reflex tests mostly the L4 nerve root; neither tests the L5 nerve root. The reliability of reflex testing can be diminished in the presence of adjacent joint or muscle problems. Up-going toes in response to stroking the plantar footpad (Babinski or plantar response) may indicate upper motor-neuron abnormalities (such as myelopathy or demyelinating disease) rather than a common low back problem.

■ *Sensory Examination.* Testing light touch or pressure in the medial (L4), dorsal (L5), and lateral (S1) aspects of the foot (Figure 1) is usually sufficient for sensory screening.

Figure 1. Testing for lumbar nerve root compromise.

Nerve root	L4	L5	S1
Pain	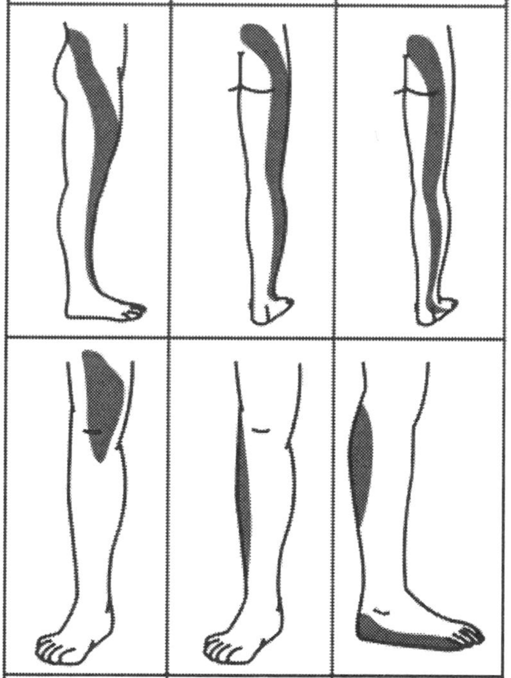		
Numbness			
Motor weakness	Extension of quadriceps.	Dorsilflexion of great toe and foot.	Plantar flexion of great toe and foot.
Screening exam	Squat & rise.	Heel walking.	Walking on toes.
Reflexes	Knee jerk diminished.	None reliable.	Ankle jerk diminished.

Clinical tests for sciatic tension

The straight leg raising (SLR) test (Figure 2) can detect tension on the L5 and/or S1 nerve root. SLR may reproduce leg pain by stretching nerve roots irritated by a disc herniation.

Figure 2. Instructions for the Straight Leg Raising (SLR) Test

(1) Ask the patient to lie as straight as possible on a table in the supine position.

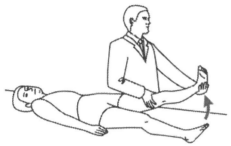

(2) With one hand placed above the knee of the leg being examined, exert enough firm pressure to keep the knee fully extended. Ask the patient to relax.

(3) With the other hand cupped under the heel, slowly raise the straight limb. Tell the patient, "If this bothers you, let me know, and I will stop."

4) Monitor for any movement of the pelvis before complaints are elicited. True sciatic tension should elicit complaints before the hamstrings are stretched enough to move the pelvis.

(5) Estimate the degree of leg elevation that elicits complaint from the patient. Then determine the most distal area of discomfort: back, hip, thigh, knee, or below the knee.

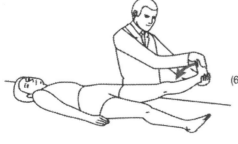

(6) While holding the leg at the limit of straight leg raising, dorsiflex the ankle. Note whether this aggravates the pain. Internal rotation of the limb can also increase the tension on the sciatic nerve roots.

Pain below the knee at less than 70 degrees of straight leg raising, aggravated by dorsiflexion of the ankle and relieved by ankle plantar flexion or external limb rotation, is most suggestive of tension on the L5 or S1 nerve root related to disc herniation. Reproducing back pain alone with SLR testing does not indicate significant nerve root tension.

Crossover pain occurs when straight raising of the patient's well limb elicits pain in the leg with sciatica. Crossover pain is a stronger indication of nerve root compression than pain elicited from raising the straight painful limb.

Sitting knee extension (Figure 3) can also test sciatic tension. The patient with significant nerve root irritation tends to complain or lean backward to reduce tension on the nerve.

Figure 3. Instructions for sitting knee extension test.

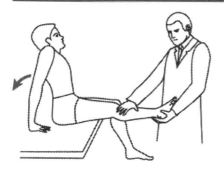

With the patient sitting on a table, both hip and knees flexed at 90 degrees, slowly extend the knee as if evaluating the patella or bottom of the foot. This maneuver stretches nerve roots as much as a moderate degree of supine SLR.

Inconsistent Findings and Pain Behavior

The patient who embellishes a medical history, exaggerates pain drawings, or provides responses on physical examination inconsistent with known physiology can be particularly challenging. A strongly positive supine straight leg raising test without complaint on sitting knee extension and inconsistent responses on examination raise a suspicion that nonphysical factors may be affecting the patient's responses. "Pain behaviors" (verbal or nonverbal communication of distress or suffering) such as amplified grimacing, distorted gait or posture, moaning, and rubbing of painful body parts may also cloud medical issues and even evoke angry responses from the clinician.

Interpreting inconsistencies or pain behaviors as malingering does not benefit the patient or the clinician. It is more useful to view such behavior and inconsistencies as the patient's attempt to enlist the practitioner as an advocate, a plea for help. The patient could be trapped in a job where activity requirements are unrealistic relative to the person's age or health. In some cases, the patient may be negotiating with an insurer or be involved in legal actions. In patients with recurrent back problems, inconsistencies and amplifications may simply be habits learned during previous medical evaluations. In working with these patients, the clinician should attempt to identify any psychological or socioeconomic pressures that might be influenced in a positive manner. The overall goal should always be to facilitate the patient's recovery and avoid the development of chronic low back disability.

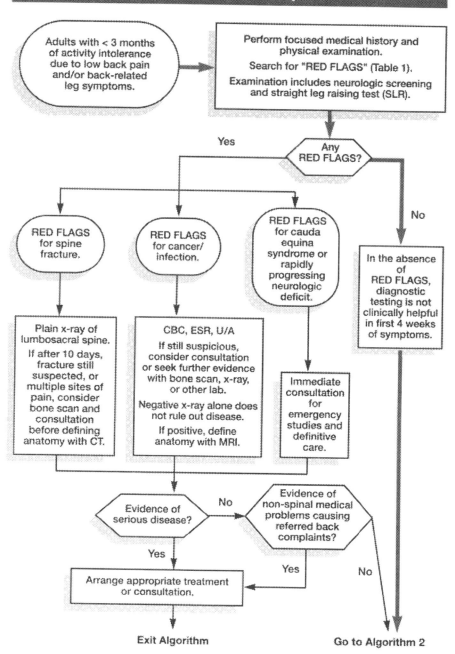

Algorithm 1.
Initial evaluation of acute low back problem

Initial Care

- Education and assurance.
- Patient comfort.
- Activity alterations.

Patient Education

If the initial assessment detects no serious condition, assure the patient that there is "no hint of a dangerous problem" and that "a rapid recovery can be expected." The need for education will vary among patients and during various stages of care. An obviously apprehensive patient may require a more detailed explanation. Patients with sciatica may have a longer expected recovery time than patients with nonspecific back symptoms and thus may need more education and reassurance. Any patient who does not recover within a few weeks may need more extensive education about back problems and the reassurance that special studies may be considered if recovery is slow.

Patient Comfort

Comfort is often a patient's first concern. Nonprescription analgesics will provide sufficient pain relief for most patients with acute low back symptoms. If treatment response is inadequate, as evidenced by continued symptoms and activity limitations, prescribed pharmaceuticals or physical methods may be added. Comorbid conditions, side effects, cost, and provider/patient preference should guide the clinician's choice of recommendations. Table 2 summarizes comfort options.

Oral Pharmaceuticals

The safest effective medication for acute low back problems appears to be acetaminophen. Nonsteroidal anti-inflammatory drugs (NSAIDs), including aspirin and ibuprofen, are also effective although they can cause gastrointestinal irritation/ulceration or (less commonly) renal or allergic problems. Phenylbutazone is not recommended due to risks of bone marrow suppression. Acetaminophen may be used safely in combination with NSAIDs or other pharmacologic or physical therapeutics, especially in otherwise healthy patients.

Muscle relaxants seem no more effective than NSAIDs for treating patients with low back symptoms, and using them in combination with NSAIDs has no demonstrated benefit. Side effects including drowsiness have been reported in up to 30 percent of patients taking muscle relaxants.

Opioids appear no more effective than safer analgesics for managing low back symptoms. Opioids should be avoided if possible and, when chosen, used only for a short time. Poor patient tolerance and risks of drowsiness, decreased reaction time, clouded judgment, and potential misuse/dependence have been reported in up to 35 percent of patients. Patients should be warned of these potentially debilitating problems.

Table 2. Symptom control methods

Recommended		
Nonprescription analgesics		
Acetaminophen (safest) NSAIDs (Aspirin,[1] Ibuprofen[1])		
Prescribed pharmaceutical methods	**Prescribed physical methods**	
Nonspecific low back symptoms and/or sciatica	**Nonspecific low back symptoms**	Sciatica
Other NSAIDs[1]	Manipulation (in place of medication or a shorter trial if combined with NSAIDs)	
Options		
Nonspecific low back symptoms and/or sciatica	**Nonspecific low back symptoms**	Sciatica
Muscle relaxants[2,3,4] Opioids[2,3,4]	Physical agents and modalities[2] (heat or cold modalities for home programs only) Shoe insoles[2]	Manipulation (in place of medication or a shorter trial if combined with NSAIDs) Physical agents and modalities[2] (heat or cold modalities for home programs only) Few days' rest[4] Shoe insoles[2]

[1] Aspirin and other NSAIDs are not recommended for use in combination with one another due to the risk of GI complications.
[2] Equivocal efficacy.
[3] Significant potential for producing drowsiness and debilitation; potential for dependency.
[4] Short course (few days only) for severe symptoms.

Physical Methods

- **Manipulation,** defined as manual loading of the spine using short or long leverage methods, is safe and effective for patients in the first month of acute low back symptoms without radiculopathy. For patients with symptoms lasting longer than 1 month, manipulation is probably safe but its efficacy is unproven. If manipulation has not resulted in symptomatic and functional improvement after 4 weeks, it should be stopped and the patient reevaluated.

- **Traction** applied to the spine has not been found effective for treating acute low back symptoms.

- **Physical modalities** such as *massage, diathermy, ultrasound, cutaneous laser treatment, biofeedback,* and *transcutaneous electrical nerve stimulation (TENS)* also have no proven efficacy in the treatment of acute low back symptoms. If requested, the clinician may wish to provide the patient with instructions on self-application of heat or cold therapy for temporary symptom relief.

- **Invasive techniques** such as *needle acupuncture* and *injection procedures* (injection of trigger points in the back; injection of facet joints; injection of steroids, lidocaine, or opioids in the epidural space) have no proven benefit in the treatment of acute low back symptoms.

- **Other miscellaneous therapies** have been evaluated. No evidence indicates that *shoe lifts* are effective in treating acute low back symptoms or limitations, especially when the difference in lower limb length is less than 2 cm. Shoe insoles are a safe and inexpensive option if requested by patients with low back symptoms who must stand for prolonged periods. Low back corsets and back belts, however, do not appear beneficial for treating acute low back symptoms.

Activity Alteration

To avoid both undue back irritation and debilitation from inactivity, recommendations for alternate activity can be helpful. Most patients will not require bed rest. Prolonged bed rest (more than 4 days) has potential debilitating effects, and its efficacy in the treatment of acute low back problems is unproven. Two to four days of bed rest are reserved for patients with the most severe limitations (due primarily to leg pain).

Avoiding undue back irritation. Activities and postures that increase stress on the back also tend to aggravate back symptoms. Patients limited by back symptoms can minimize the stress of lifting by keeping any lifted object close to the body at the level of the navel. Twisting, bending, and reaching while lifting also increase stress on the back. Sitting, although safe, may aggravate symptoms for some patients. Advise these patients to avoid prolonged sitting and to change position often. A soft support placed at the small of the back, armrests to support some body weight, and a slight recline of the chair back may make required sitting more comfortable.

Avoiding debilitation. Until the patient returns to normal activity, aerobic (endurance) conditioning exercise such as walking, stationary biking, swimming, and even light jogging may be recommended to help avoid debilitation from inactivity. An incremental, gradually increasing regimen of aerobic exercise (up to 20 to 30 minutes daily) can usually be started within the first 2 weeks of symptoms. Such conditioning activities have been found to stress the back no more than sitting for an equal time period on the side of the bed. Patients should be informed that exercise may increase symptoms slightly at first. If intolerable, some exercise alteration is usually helpful.

Conditioning exercises for trunk muscles are more mechanically stressful to the back than aerobic exercise. Such exercises are not recommended during the first few weeks of symptoms, although they may later help patients regain and maintain activity tolerance.

There is no evidence to indicate that back-specific exercise machines are effective for treating acute low back problems. Neither is there evidence that stretching of the back helps patients with acute symptoms.

Work Activities

When requested, clinicians may choose to offer specific instructions about activity at work for patients with acute limitations due to low back symptoms. The patient's age, general health, and perceptions of safe limits of sitting, standing, walking or lifting (noted on initial history) can help provide reasonable starting points for activity recommendations. Table 3 provides a guide for recommendations about sitting and lifting. The clinician should make clear to patients and employers that:

- Even moderately heavy unassisted lifting may aggravate back symptoms.

- Any restrictions are intended to allow for spontaneous recovery or time to build activity tolerance through exercise.

Activity restrictions are prescribed for a short time period only, depending upon work requirements (no benefits apparent beyond 3 months).

Table 3. Guidelines for sitting and unassisted lifting

	Symptoms					
	Severe	→	Moderate	→	Mild	→	None
Sitting[1]	20 min	→	→	→	→	→	50 min
Unassisted lifting[2]						
Men	20 lbs	→	20 lbs	→	60 lbs	→	80 lbs
Women	20 lbs	→	20 lbs	→	35 lbs	→	40 lbs

[1]Without getting up and moving around.
[2]Modification of NIOSH Lifting Guidelines, 1981, 1993. Gradually increase unassisted lifting limits to 60 lbs (men) and 35 lbs (women) by 3 months even with continued symptoms. Instruct patient to limit twisting, bending, reaching while lifting and to hold lifted object as close to navel as possible.

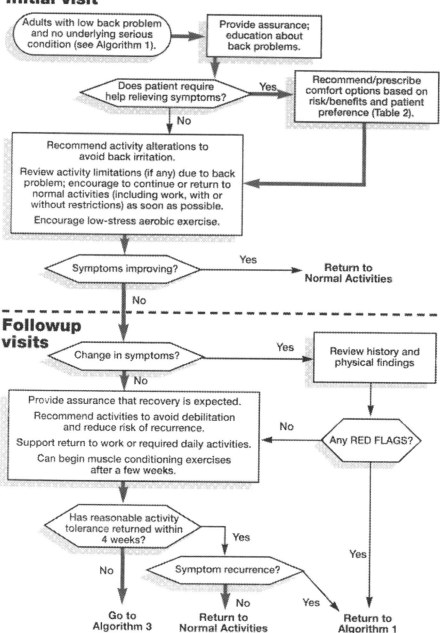

Algorithm 2. Treatment of acute low back problem on initial and followup visits

Initial visit

Adults with low back problem and no underlying serious condition (see Algorithm 1).

Provide assurance; education about back problems.

Does patient require help relieving symptoms?

Yes → Recommend/prescribe comfort options based on risk/benefits and patient preference (Table 2).

No

Recommend activity alterations to avoid back irritation.

Review activity limitations (if any) due to back problem; encourage to continue or return to normal activities (including work, with or without restrictions) as soon as possible.

Encourage low-stress aerobic exercise.

Symptoms improving?

Yes → **Return to Normal Activities**

No

Followup visits

Change in symptoms?

Yes → Review history and physical findings

No

Provide assurance that recovery is expected.

Recommend activities to avoid debilitation and reduce risk of recurrence.

Support return to work or required daily activities.

Can begin muscle conditioning exercises after a few weeks.

Any RED FLAGS?

No

Has reasonable activity tolerance returned within 4 weeks?

Yes → Symptom recurrence?

No

Go to Algorithm 3

No → **Return to Normal Activities**

Yes

Yes → **Return to Algorithm 1**

Special Studies and Diagnostic Considerations

Routine testing (laboratory tests, plain x-rays of the lumbosacral spine) and imaging studies are not recommended during the first month of activity limitation due to back symptoms except when a red flag noted on history or examination raises suspicion of a dangerous low back or non-spinal condition. If a patient's limitations due to low back symptoms do not improve in 4 weeks, reassessment is recommended. After again reviewing the patient's activity limitations, history, and physical findings, the clinician may then consider further diagnostic studies, and discuss these with the patient.

Timing and Limits of Special Studies

Waiting 4 weeks before considering special tests allows 90 percent of patients to recover spontaneously and avoids unneeded procedures. This also reduces the potential confusion of falsely labeling age-related changes on imaging studies (commonly noted in patients older than 30 without back symptoms) as the cause of the acute symptoms. In the absence of either red flags or persistent activity limitations due to continuous limb symptoms, imaging studies (especially plain x-rays) rarely provide information that changes the clinical approach to the acute low back problem.

Selection of Special Studies

Prior to ordering imaging studies the clinician should have noted either of the following:

■ The emergence of a red flag.

■ Physiologic evidence of tissue insult or neurologic dysfunction.

Physiologic evidence may be in the form of definitive nerve findings on physical examination, electrodiagnostic studies (when evaluating sciatica), and a laboratory test or bone scan (when evaluating nonspecific low back symptoms). Unquestionable findings that identify specific nerve root compromise on the neurologic examination (see Figure 1) are sufficient physiologic evidence to warrant imaging. When the neurologic examination is less clear, however, further physiologic evidence of nerve root dysfunction should be considered before ordering an imaging study. Electromyography (EMG) including H-reflex tests may be useful to identify subtle focal neurologic dysfunction in patients with leg symptoms lasting longer than 3-4 weeks. Sensory evoked potentials (SEPs) may be added to the assessment if spinal stenosis or spinal cord myelopathy is suspected.

Laboratory tests such as erythrocyte sedimentation rate (ESR), complete blood count (CBC), and urinalysis (UA) can be useful to screen for nonspecific medical diseases (especially infection and tumor) of the low back. A bone scan can detect physiologic reactions to suspected spinal tumor, infection, or occult fracture.

Should physiologic evidence indicate tissue insult or nerve impairment, discuss with a consultant selection of an imaging test to define a potential anatomic cause (CT for bone, MRI for neural or other soft tissue). Anatomic definition is commonly needed to guide surgery or specific procedures. Selection of an imaging test should also take into consideration any patient allergies to contrast media (myelogram) or concerns about claustrophobia (MRI) and costs. A discussion with a specialist on selection of the most clinically valuable study can often assist the primary care clinician to avoid duplication. Table 4 provides a general comparison of the abilities of different techniques to identify physiologic insult and define anatomic defects. Missing from the table is discography, which is not recommended for assessing patients with acute low back symptoms.

In general, an imaging study may be an appropriate consideration for the patient whose limitations due to consistent symptoms have persisted for 1 month or more:

■ When surgery is being considered for treatment of a specific detectable loss of neurologic function.

■ To further evaluate potentially serious spinal pathology.

Reliance upon imaging studies alone to evaluate the source of low back symptoms, however, carries a significant risk of diagnostic confusion, given the possibility of falsely identifying a finding that was present before symptoms began.

Table 4. Ability of different techniques to identify and define pathology

Technique	Identify physiologic insult	Define anatomic defect
History	+	+
Physical examination:		
Circumference measurements	+	+
Reflexes	++	++
Straight leg raising (SLR)	++	+
Crossed SLR	+++	++
Motor	++	++
Sensory	++	++
Laboratory studies (ESR, CBC, UA)	++	0
Bone scan[1]	+++	++
EMG/SEP	+++	++
X-ray[1]	0	+
CT[1]	0	++++[2]
MRI	0	++++[2]
Myelo-CT[1]	0	++++[2]
Myelography[1]	0	++++[2]

[1] Risk of complications (radiation, infection, etc.): highest for myelo-CT, second highest for myelography, and relatively less risk for bone scan, x-ray, and CT.

[2] False-positive diagnostic findings in up to 30 percent of people without symptoms at age 30.

Note: Number of plus signs indicates relative ability to identify or define.

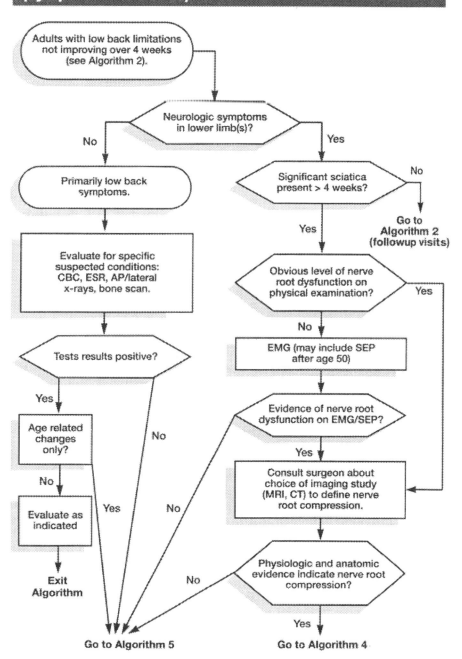

Algorithm 3. Evaluation of the slow-to-recover patient (symptoms > 4 weeks)

Adults with low back limitations not improving over 4 weeks (see Algorithm 2).

Neurologic symptoms in lower limb(s)?

No — Primarily low back symptoms.

Evaluate for specific suspected conditions: CBC, ESR, AP/lateral x-rays, bone scan.

Tests results positive?

Yes — Age related changes only?

No — Evaluate as indicated

Exit Algorithm

Yes / No — Go to Algorithm 5

Yes — Significant sciatica present > 4 weeks?

No — Go to Algorithm 2 (followup visits)

Yes — Obvious level of nerve root dysfunction on physical examination?

No — EMG (may include SEP after age 50)

Evidence of nerve root dysfunction on EMG/SEP?

Yes — Consult surgeon about choice of imaging study (MRI, CT) to define nerve root compression.

Yes — (from Obvious level of nerve root dysfunction)

Physiologic and anatomic evidence indicate nerve root compression?

No — Go to Algorithm 5

Yes — Go to Algorithm 4

Management Considerations After Special Studies

Definitive treatment for serious conditions (see Table 1) detected by special studies is beyond the scope of this guideline. When special studies fail to define the exact cause of symptoms, however, no patient should receive an impression that the clinician thinks "nothing is wrong" or that the problem could be "in their head." Assure the patient that a clinical workup is highly successful in detecting serious conditions, but does not reveal the precise cause of most low back symptoms.

Surgical Considerations

Within the first 3 months of acute low back symptoms, surgery is considered only when serious spinal pathology or nerve root dysfunction obviously due to a herniated lumbar disc is detected. A disc herniation, characterized by protrusion of the central nucleus pulposus through a defect in the outer annulus fibrosis, may trap a nerve root causing irritation, leg symptoms and nerve root dysfunction. The presence of a herniated lumbar disc on an imaging study, however, does not necessarily imply nerve root dysfunction. Studies of asymptomatic adults commonly demonstrate intervertebral disc herniations that apparently do not entrap a nerve root or cause symptoms.

Therefore, nerve root decompression can be considered for a patient if all of the following criteria exist:

- Sciatica is both severe and disabling.

- Symptoms of sciatica persist without improvement for longer than 4 weeks or with extreme progression.

- There is strong physiologic evidence of dysfunction of a specific nerve root with intervertebral disc herniation confirmed at the corresponding level and side by findings on an imaging study.

Patients with acute low back pain alone, without findings of serious conditions or significant nerve root compression, rarely benefit from a surgical consultation.

Many patients with strong clinical findings of nerve root dysfunction due to disc herniation recover activity tolerance within 1 month; no evidence indicates that delaying surgery for this period worsens outcomes. With or without an operation, more than 80 percent of patients with obvious surgical indications eventually recover. Surgery seems to be a luxury for speeding recovery of patients with obvious surgical indications but benefits fewer than 40 percent of patients with questionable physiologic findings. Moreover, surgery increases the chance of future procedures with higher complication rates. Overall, the incidence of first-time disc surgery complications, including infection and bleeding, is less than 1 percent. The figure increases dramatically with older patients or repeated procedures.

Direct and indirect nerve root decompression for herniated discs. Direct methods of nerve root decompression include laminotomy (expansion of the interlaminar space for access to the nerve root and the offending disc fragments), microdiscectomy (laminotomy using a microscope), and laminectomy (total removal of laminae). Methods of indirect nerve root decompression include chemonucleolysis, the injection of chymopapain or other enzymes to dissolve the inner disc. Such chemical treatment methods are less efficacious than standard or microdiscectomy and have rare but serious complications. Any of these methods is preferable to percutaneous discectomy (indirect, mechanical disc removal through a lateral disc puncture).

Management of spinal stenosis. Usually resulting from soft tissue and bony encroachment of the spinal canal and nerve roots, spinal stenosis typically has a gradual onset and begins in older adults. It is characterized by nonspecific limb symptoms, called *neurogenic claudication* or *pseudoclaudication,* that interfere with the duration of comfortable standing and walking. The symptoms are commonly bilateral and rarely associated with strong focal findings on examination.

Neurogenic claudication, however, can be confused or coexist with *vascular claudication,* in which leg pain also limits walking. The symptoms of vascular insufficiency can be relieved by simply standing still while relief of neurogenic claudication symptoms usually require the patient to flex the lumbar spine or sit.

The surgical treatment for spinal stenosis is usually complete laminectomy for posterior decompression. Offending soft tissue and osteophytes that encroach upon nerve roots in the central spinal canal and foramen are removed. Fusion may be considered to stabilize a degenerative spondylolisthesis with motion between the slipped vertebra and adjacent vertebrae. Elderly patients with spinal stenosis who tolerate their daily activities usually need no surgery unless they develop new signs of bowel or bladder dysfunction. Decisions on treatment should take into account the patient's preference, lifestyle, other medical problems, and risks of surgery. Surgery for spinal stenosis is rarely considered in the first 3 months of symptoms.

Except for cases of trauma-related spinal fracture or dislocation, fusion alone is not usually considered in the first 3 months following onset of low back symptoms.

Algorithm 4. Surgical considerations for patients with persistent sciatica

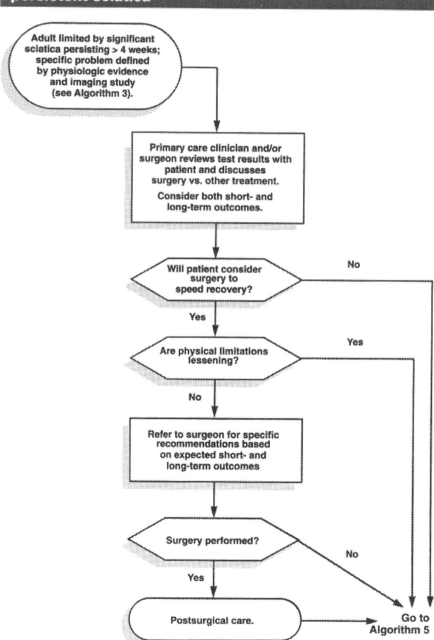

Adult limited by significant sciatica persisting > 4 weeks; specific problem defined by physiologic evidence and imaging study (see Algorithm 3).

Primary care clinician and/or surgeon reviews test results with patient and discusses surgery vs. other treatment.

Consider both short- and long-term outcomes.

Will patient consider surgery to speed recovery?

No

Yes

Are physical limitations lessening?

Yes

No

Refer to surgeon for specific recommendations based on expected short- and long-term outcomes

Surgery performed?

No

Yes

Postsurgical care.

Go to Algorithm 5

Further Management Considerations

Following diagnostic or surgical procedures, the management of most patients becomes focused on improving physical conditioning through an incrementally increased exercise program. The goal of this program is to build activity tolerance and overcome individual limitations due to back symptoms. At this point in treatment, symptom control methods are only an adjunct to making prescribed exercises more tolerable.

■ Begin with low-stress aerobic activities to improve general stamina (walking, riding a bicycle, swimming, and eventually jogging).

■ Exercises to condition specific trunk muscles can be added a few weeks after. The back muscles may need to be in better condition than before the problem occurred. Otherwise, the back may continue to be painful and easily irritated by even mild activity. Following back surgery, recovery of activity tolerance may be delayed until protective muscles are conditioned well enough to compensate for any remaining structural changes.

■ Finally, specific training to perform activities required at home or work can begin. The objective of this program is to increase the patient's tolerance in carrying out actual daily duties.

When patients demonstrate difficulty regaining the ability to tolerate the activities they are required (or would like) to do, the clinician may pose the following diagnostic and treatment questions:

■ Could the patient have a serious, undetected medical condition? A careful review of the medical history and physical examination is warranted.

■ Are the patient's activity goals realistic? Exploring briefly the patient's expectations, both short- and long-term, of being able to perform specific activities at home, work, or recreation may help the patient assess whether such activity levels are actually achievable.

■ If for any reason the achievement of activity goals seems unlikely, what are the patient's remaining options? To answer this question, the patient is often required to gather specific information from family, friends, employers, or others. If, on followup visits, the patient has made no effort to gather such information, the clinician has the opportunity to point out that low back symptoms alone rarely prevent a patient from addressing questions so important to his or her future. This observation can lead to an open, nonjudgmental discussion of common but complicated psychosocial problems or other issues that often can interfere with a patient's recovery from low back problems. The clinician can then help the patient address or arrange further evaluation of any specific problem limiting the patient's progress. This can usually be accomplished as the patient continues, with the clinician's encouragement, to build activity tolerance through safe, simple exercises.

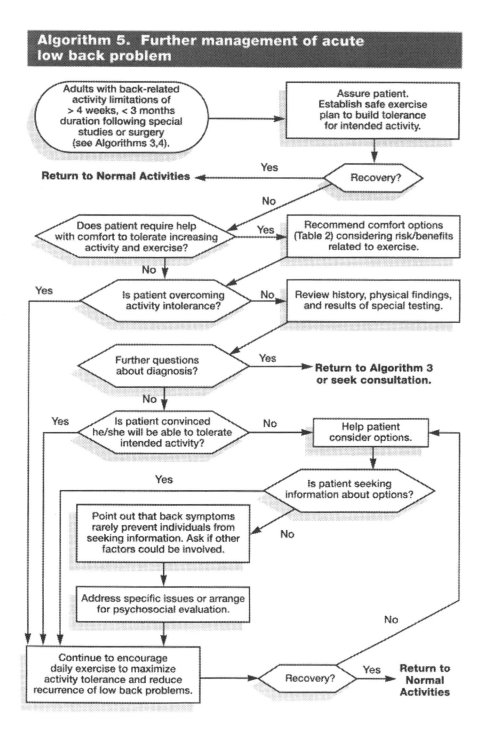

Algorithm 5. Further management of acute low back problem

Adults with back-related activity limitations of > 4 weeks, < 3 months duration following special studies or surgery (see Algorithms 3,4).

Assure patient. Establish safe exercise plan to build tolerance for intended activity.

Recovery? → Yes → **Return to Normal Activities**

No

Does patient require help with comfort to tolerate increasing activity and exercise? → Yes → Recommend comfort options (Table 2) considering risk/benefits related to exercise.

No

Is patient overcoming activity intolerance? → No → Review history, physical findings, and results of special testing.

Yes

Further questions about diagnosis? → Yes → **Return to Algorithm 3 or seek consultation.**

No

Is patient convinced he/she will be able to tolerate intended activity? → No → Help patient consider options.

Yes

Is patient seeking information about options?

Point out that back symptoms rarely prevent individuals from seeking information. Ask if other factors could be involved. ← No

Address specific issues or arrange for psychosocial evaluation.

Continue to encourage daily exercise to maximize activity tolerance and reduce recurrence of low back problems. → Recovery? → Yes → **Return to Normal Activities**

No

Table 5. Summary of Guideline Recommendations

The ratings in parentheses indicate the scientific evidence supporting each recommendation according to the following scale:

A = strong research-based evidence (multiple relevant and high-quality scientific studies).

B = moderate research-based evidence (one relevant, high-quality scientific study or multiple adequate scientific studies).

C = limited research-based evidence (at least one adequate scientific study in patients with low back pain).

D = panel interpretation of evidence not meeting inclusion criteria for research-based evidence.

The number of studies meeting panel review criteria is noted for each category.

	Recommend	Option	Recommend against
History and physical exam 34 studies	Basic history (B). History of cancer/infection (B). Signs/symptoms of cauda equina syndrome (C). History of significant trauma (C). Psychosocial history (C). Straight leg raising test (B). Focused neurological exam (B).	Pain drawing and visual analog scale(D).	
Patient education 14 studies	Patient education about low back symptoms (B). Back school in occupational settings (C).	Back school in non-occupational settings (C).	
Medication 23 studies	Acetaminophen (C). NSAIDs (B).	Muscle relaxants (C). Opioids, short course (C).	Opioids used >2 wks (C). Phenylbutazone (C). Oral steroids (C). Colchicine (B). Antidepressants (C).
Physical treatment methods 42 studies	Manipulation of low back during first month of symptoms (B).	Manipulation for patients with radiculopathy (C). Manipulation for patients with symptoms >1 month (C). Self-application of heat or cold to low back. Shoe insoles (C). Corset for prevention in occupational setting (C).	Manipulation for patients with undiagnosed neurologic deficits (D). Prolonged course of manipulation (D). Traction (B). TENS (C). Biofeedback (C). Shoe lifts (D). Corset for treatment (D).
Injections 26 studies		Epidural steroid injections for radicular pain to avoid surgery (C).	Epidural injections for back pain without radiculopathy (D). Trigger point injections (C). Ligamentous injections (C). Facet joint injections (C). Needle acupuncture (D).

	Recommend	Option	Recommend against
Bed rest 4 studies		Bed rest of 2-4 days for severe radiulopathy (D).	Bed rest > 4 days (B).
Activities and exercise 20 studies	Temporary avoidance of activities that increase mechanical stress on spine (D). Gradual return to normal activities (B). Low-stress aerobic exercise (C). Conditioning exercises for trunk muscles after 2 weeks (C). Exercise quotas (C).		Back-specific exercise machines (D). Therapeutic stretching of back muscles (D).
Detection of physiologic abnormalities 14 studies	If no improvement after 1 month, consider: Bone scan (C). Needle EMG and H-reflex tests to clarify nerve root dysfunction (C). SEP to assess spinal stenosis (C).		EMG for clinically obvious radiculopathy (D). Surface EMG and F-wave tests (C). Thermography (C).
X-rays of L-S spine 18 studies	When red flags for fracture present (C). When red flags for cancer or infection present (C).		Routine use in first month of symptoms in absence of red flags (B). Routine oblique views (B).
Imaging 18 studies	CT or MRI when cauda equina, tumor, infection, or fracture strongly suspected (C). MRI test of choice for patients with prior back surgery (D). Assure quality criteria for imaging tests (B).	Myelography or CT-myelography for preoperative planning (D).	Use of imaging test before one month in absence red flags (B). Discography or CT-discography (C).
Surgical considerations 14 studies	Discuss surgical options with patients with persistent and severe sciatica and clinical evidence of nerve root compromise after 1 month of conservative therapy (B). Standard discectomy and microdiscectomy of similar efficacy in treatment of herniated disc (B). Chymopapain, used after ruling out allergic sensitivity, acceptable but less efficacious than discectomy to treat herniated disc (C).		Disc surgery in patients with back pain alone, no red flags, and no nerve root compression (D). Percutaneous discectomy less efficacious than chymopapain (C). Surgery for spinal stenosis within the first 3 months of symptoms (D). Stenosis surgery when justified by imaging test rather than patient's functional status (D). Spinal fusion during the first 3 months of symptoms in the absence of fracture, dislocation, complications of tumor or infection (C).
Psychosocial factors	Social, economic, and psychological factors can alter patient response to symptoms and treatment (D).		Referral for extensive evaluation/treatment prior to exploring patient expectations or psychosocial factors (D).

Appendix D

Glossary

Some of the terms in this glossary have more than one definition or are used ambiguously by chiropractors. The definitions below are consistent with the use of these terms throughout this book and reflect what chiropractors usually mean.

Activator Adjusting Instrument. A handheld instrument used by chiropractors who assert that slightly misaligned vertebrae can be tapped back into place with a mallet.

Acupressure. A method of applying manual or instrument pressure to acupuncture points as a treatment for illness, addiction, and other problems. Among chiropractors, acupressure is more popular than acupuncture.

Acupuncture. Puncturing the skin with needles, based on mystical notions that stimulating certain "acupoints" along hypothetical channels ("meridians") in the skin will influence certain organs. Although acupuncture may be effective in relieving some types of pain, there is no reason to believe that it is effective in the treatment of disease. Some chiropractors use acupuncture or acupressure, along with spinal adjustments, to treat a variety of ailments.

Acute back pain. Back pain that lasts a short while, usually a few days to several weeks. Episodes lasting longer than three months are not considered acute.

"Alternative" health care. Misleading term used to characterize many types of unscientific methods. Since ineffective methods are not true alternatives to effective ones, the terms "unscientific" or "dubious" are more appropriate.

AMA. Abbreviation for American Medical Association, which is organized medicine's largest group.

American Chiropractic Association (ACA). The largest chiropractic association, representing "mixer" chiropractors who combine physical therapy and other nondrug methods with spinal adjustments.

Ankylosing spondylitis. Arthritis of the spine, an inflammatory disease that causes spinal joints to fuse (ankylose).

Applied kinesiology. An unscientific method of testing muscle strength to detect the presence of disease, vitamin deficiency, and other problems.

Articular. Pertaining to a joint.

Articulation (of bones). Synonym for "joint."

ASC. Abbreviation for "atlas subluxation complex," which some chiropractors feel is the most common and the most serious vertebral misalignment. Chiropractors who practice specific "upper cervical techniques" focus on the ASC.

Atlas. Topmost vertebra of the neck.

Atlas orthogonal technique (A.O.T.). One of many methods of correcting cervical "subluxations" claimed to be responsible for problems anywhere in the body.

Autonomic nervous system. The part of the nervous system that helps control many of the body's automatic processes, such as blood pressure maintenance. It includes the sympathetic and parasympathetic nerves, which are described below.

Ayurvedic medicine. A system of natural healing (from India) with the goal of bringing humans into harmony or equilibrium with their environment. Diet, medication, herbs, and other measures are used to cleanse the mind and body and to improve health. Some chiropractors include ayurvedic medicine in holistic healing programs.

Barge analysis. A contemporary technique, developed by a straight chiropractor, used to locate alleged shifting of a disk nucleus said to cause tortipelvis/ torticollis, spinal distortions, or curvatures. Rotation of a spinous process toward the wide side of a disk space on the concave side of a spinal curve (the opposite of what is normally seen) is thought to indicate that the disk is improperly centered.

"Big Idea." The chiropractic concept that the body heals itself when interference to the proper functioning of the nervous system is removed.

Bio Energetic Synchronization Technique (B.E.S.T.). A nonsensical method that involves measuring leg length to determine whether "imbalances" exist in the body's electromagnetic field. The chiropractor allegedly corrects these imbalances by placing his hands on certain "contact points" to transfer electromagnetic energy to the patient.

Bio-kinetics. A new technique in which a special adjustment with an instrument is made between the atlas and the skull to relieve dozens of ailments ranging from asthma to psoriasis. This cure-all spinal adjustment corrects subluxations and "reconstructs the spine."

Blair upper cervical technique. Another technique that concentrates upon correction of vertebral misalignments at the top of the neck as a method of removing nerve interference in the spine. A "Blair head clamp" is used to position the head for cervical x-ray examination.

Bone scan. Image of bone produced on film after the patient is given an intravenous injection of radioactive material that accumulates in areas of diseased or injured bone.

Bonesetters. Term used years ago to describe nonmedical and often professionally untrained individuals who learned or developed the skill of reducing dislocated joints. Spinal manipulation is believed to have been included in the ancient art of bonesetting.

C.A. Abbreviation for "chiropractic assistant." Training for this position is usually done on-the-job but is available at some chiropractic colleges.

Carver technique. Method developed by Willard Carver, an early Palmer student who formulated his own theories about subluxations and nerve interference and opened the Carver Chiropractic college in 1908. Carver developed a technique in which traction and pressure is applied to the spine just before making a manual thrust, which he called the "Tracto-Thrust" system.

Cauda equina syndrome. A group of signs and symptoms that can occur when nerves near the lower end of the spine are defective or damaged. The symptoms include weakness of the legs, loss of feeling in the perineal area (saddle anesthesia), and loss of control of the bladder or bowels. The problem can be due to a birth defect or to protrusion of a lumbar disk into the spinal canal.

Cavitation. Pop that occurs in a spinal joint when vertebral surfaces (facets) are separated to create a vacuum that pulls in nitrogen gas.

Cerebrovascular accident (CVA). Stroke.

Cervical vertebrae. There are seven vertebrae in the cervical or neck area of the spine.

Chelation therapy. Intravenous administration of a synthetic amino acid (EDTA) to "clean out the arteries." While such treatment can be effective in removing such heavy metals as lead from the body, there is no evidence that it is effective against arterial disease. Although chiropractors are not licensed to perform chelation therapy, some "integrated" holistic chiropractic clinics employ a medical doctor to perform this procedure.

Chiropractic biophysics. Method of chiropractic analysis and treatment in which spinal corrections are based on "mathematics and physics" rather than on anatomical considerations. This technique advocates forced cervical extension to develop a "normal neck curve." However, it is normal for some persons to have a cervical curve that deviates from what is considered "normal."

Chronic back pain. Back pain episode that lasts more than three months.

Coccyx. The "tailbone" in the buttock area at the bottom of the spine—an evolutionary remnant of the tail present in lower species of animals.

Complementary care. Healthcare practice purported to combine standard and "alternative" approaches.

Computerized axial tomography (also called CAT scan or CT scan). Imaging method in which the density of an area of the body is determined by passing x-rays fed into a computer to create a picture on a screen similar to a cross-sectional photograph.

Concept therapy. Method of using a positive state of mind to help "innate intelligence" heal the body, thus making any chiropractic technique more effective. Its founder taught that once you know the "great secret" taught in Concept Therapy, you can make any technique work.

Contact Reflex Analysis (CRA). A nonsensical testing procedure in which diagnoses are made by testing muscle strength while placing manual pressure on alleged "reflex points." The results are then used to prescribe vitamin supplements and/or homeopathic products.

Contour analysis. Useless procedure in which an angled light is passed through a grid to the surface of the patient's body to produce a pattern of shadows that is viewed on a screen and/or photographed. The resultant picture resembles a topographic map. Also called moire contourographic analysis.

Contraindication. Reason that diagnostic or treatment procedures might be dangerous and therefore should not be used. Nerve damage caused by a herniated disk, for example, may contraindicate spinal manipulation.

Cox flexion-distraction technique. Method of applying manually controlled distraction or stretching to specific spinal segments with the assistance of a movable table. Not a manipulation technique.

Cult. Any system that encourages obsessive devotion to a person or an ideal.

D.C. Abbreviation for "doctor of chiropractic."

D.C.M. (Doctor of Chiropractic Medicine). New degree being considered by at least one chiropractic college, which believes that some form of drug therapy may be appropriate for a properly specialized chiropractic practice.

Derefield leg check. Test alleged to detect pelvic dysfunction by measuring leg length in a prone (facedown) position. Measurements are obtained with the legs straight and with the knees bent. Leg checks are used by Activator practitioners and others who purport to measure and correct pelvic "imbalances."

Directional nonforce technique (DNFT). Method of diagnosing and correcting subluxations by applying thumb pressure to the spine and checking leg length, which supposedly changes when correction is made.

Disk degeneration. Deterioration of disk cartilage as a result of wear and tear or disk herniation. Osteophyte (spur) formation may occur as part of the process

D.O. Abbreviation for "doctor of osteopathy."

Dynamic thrust. Chiropractic adjustment delivered suddenly and forcefully to move vertebrae, often resulting in a popping sound.

Enzyme (oral). Protein substance that triggers and speeds up (catalyzes) chemical reactions within the body. Oral enzymes, usually obtained from plants, are typically marketed with false claims that they will remedy "enzyme-deficient" diets. However, when taken by mouth, they are digested and do not influence the body's metabolic reactions.

Enzyme replacement system. Nonsensical approach that correlates recurring "subluxation patterns" with the results of a 24-hour urinalysis (purported to identify "enzyme deficiencies") so that spinal adjustments and nutritional measures can be combined.

Facets. Bony surfaces that form joints between the vertebrae.

Federation of Straight Chiropractors and Organizations (FSCO). Organization representing super-straight chiropractors who assert that vertebral subluxation is the primary cause of disease and that spinal adjustment is the most important treatment.

Flexion-distraction technique. Useful method of stretching the spine in a facedown position on a table that allows manually applied flexion and traction to be applied to specific spinal segments.

"Four stages of spinal degeneration." An alleged progressive degeneration of the spine that some chiropractors claim occurs when symptomless vertebral subluxations remain uncorrected. Some chiropractors use this to motivate patients to come for "maintenance" care.

Full-spine technique. Method of adjusting or manipulating any of the vertebrae from the neck down.

Gonstead technique. System of correcting pelvic and sacral "subluxations" to correct secondary subluxations elsewhere in the spine. The alleged problem areas are located by motion palpation and skin-temperature instrument measurement and "confirmed" with full-spine x-ray examination.

Grostic procedure. Upper cervical technique that depends upon x-ray examination to measure and detect misalignments between the atlas and the skull. Adjustment can be made with an instrument or be done manually by placing pressure on the side of the neck at the base of the skull.

Herniated disk. Rupture of an intervertebral disk with protrusion of disk cartilage from between the vertebrae.

Hole-in-One (H.I.O.). Method of adjusting the atlas (the topmost vertebra at the base of the skull). Proponents claim that this will improve health and facilitate correction of subluxations elsewhere in the spine.

Homeopathy. Pseudoscientific system that uses highly diluted solutions made from substances said to produce the same symptoms of the disease being treated.

ICA Review. The bimonthly journal of the International Chiropractors Association, a "straight" chiropractic organization.

Informed consent. Permission given by a patient who has been fully apprised of the nature and risks of a proposed treatment.

Innate Intelligence. An alleged inborn ability of the body to heal itself, which chiropractors believe is enhanced by spinal adjustments.

Intermittent claudication. Consistent cramping of muscles in one or both legs after walking a certain distance, caused by an oxygen debt resulting from circulatory insufficiency. Symptoms are quickly relieved with rest.

International Chiropractors Association (ICA). The second-largest chiropractic association, representing "'straight" chiropractors who feel that spinal adjustment is the most important treatment for disease.

Intervertebral disk. The tough cartilage that serves as a cushion between two vertebrae. Each disk has a gelatinous-like center (nucleus pulposus) that may protrude to form a disk herniation.

JACA. Abbreviation for the monthly *Journal of the American Chiropractic Association*, which reflects the beliefs of the majority of chiropractors.

JMPT. Abbreviation for the *Journal of Manipulative and Physiological Therapeutics*, published nine times a year by the National College of Chiropractic and "Dedicated to the Advancement of Chiropractic Health Care Principles and Practice." It is peer-reviewed and listed in the *Index Medicus*.

JNMS. Abbreviation for the *Journal of the Neuromusculoskeletal System*, a sensible, specialized peer-reviewed journal dealing with the diagnosis and treatment of neuromusculoskeletal problems. It is published quarterly by the American Chiropractic Association.

Kale method. Variety of upper cervical adjustment in which a "toggle adjustment," or a sudden, shallow thrust is applied to the side of the neck to correct atlas subluxations, often in a knee-chest position on a special table.

"Killer subluxations." Allegedly misaligned spinal bones that some chiropractors feel can result in fatal illness. The concept is promoted by posters that depict an unrealistically large spinal nerve being pinched by an unrealistically displaced vertebra.

Kyphosis. Abnormal rearward curvature of the thoracic spine that results in a hump. Also called hunchback.

L.Ac. Abbreviation for "licensed acupuncturist."

Leander's method. Method that utilizes a motorized table for loosening or mobilizing the spine with flexion-distraction-type stretching before a spinal adjustment.

Leg-length testing. An unsubstantiated method used to detect alleged subluxations. It is used as part of Activator Methods, Logan basic, Bio Energetic Synchronization Technique, Thompson terminal point technique, and Sacro occipital technique.

Listing. Abbreviated description of the position or movement of a "subluxated" vertebra. Many techniques have their own listing system, which can make it difficult for chiropractors to communicate with each other.

Locked spinal joint. Sudden binding that occurs when two joint surfaces are shifted out of their normal alignment by an awkward movement that triggers muscle spasm. The result may also be called an "acute locked back."

Logan basic. A nonthrusting method in which thumb pressure is used to correct alleged sacral subluxations and leg deficiency claimed to affect the entire spine.

Long-lever manipulation. Method of spinal manipulation in which a general technique is used to stretch or loosen several vertebrae at a time.

Low-force technique. Use of an adjusting machine and/or reflex technique said to be an alternative to forceful manipulation ("dynamic thrust"). It may not be an appropriate substitute for properly performed spinal manipulation. Advertising it is often a promotion gimmick.

Lumbar vertebrae. The five bones in the lower-back portion of the spine.

Lumbo-pelvic techniques. Technique used to adjust any "manipulative lesion" in the joints of the lumbar spine and pelvis. Lumbo-pelvic "distortions" are attributed to postural alterations, leg-length inequality, tilting of the lumbar vertebrae, loss of mobility, and other "lesions" that require manipulation over the pelvis and lower back. Leg-length testing is often used to detect lumbo-pelvic distortions.

Lumbosacral strain. Strain or injury of joints or ligaments at the base of the spine where the last lumbar vertebra (L5) is connected to the sacrum. Strain or disk degeneration in this area is probably the most common cause of low-back pain.

Magnetic resonance imaging (MRI). A method of using the energy of a magnetic field to obtain cross-sectional images of body structures. No radiation is involved.

Maintenance care. Subluxation-based program of periodic spinal examinations and "adjustments" alleged to help maintain the patient's health. Also called "preventive maintenance" or "preventative maintenance."

Managed care. Health-care system (such as HMO or PPO) that integrates the financing and delivery of services by using selected providers, utilization review, and financial incentives for members who use the providers and procedures authorized by the plan.

Manipulation under anesthesia (MUA). Procedure in which a chiropractor performs manipulation while an anesthesiologist keeps the patient asleep. MUA has little appropriate use and is potentially dangerous. Because the normal protective reflexes are abolished, the manipulated joint can be overstretched.

Mercy Guidelines. Common name for the report issued following the chiropractic consensus conference held at the Mercy Conference Center in Burlingame, California, on January 25–30, 1992. The report is a step toward establishing parameters and guidelines for the profession. Many insurance companies use it as a guide to the appropriateness of chiropractic treatment.

Meric system. Chiropractic system based on the theory that specific spinal joints are associated with specific organs, requiring adjustment of certain vertebrae for certain diseases.

Meridian therapy. Term that encompasses acupuncture, acupressure, and other techniques purported to balance the flow of the body's "life force" by stimulating various points (acupoints) located throughout the body.

"Mixer." Chiropractor who uses physical therapy and other natural treatment methods in addition to manual manipulation of the spine.

Mobilization. Method of manipulation, movement, or stretching to increase range of motion in muscles and joints that does not involve a high-velocity thrust.

Moire contourographic analysis. See **Contour analysis.**

Motion palpation. Useful method of locating fixations and loss of mobility in the spine by feeling the motion of specific spinal segments as the patient moves.

Musculoskeletal. Referring to structures involving tendons, muscles, ligaments, and joints.

Myofascitis. Inflammation of muscle fibers and their surrounding sheaths.

N.D. Abbreviation for "doctor of naturopathy."

National Association for Chiropractic Medicine (NACM). A small group of reformist chiropractors who have denounced the chiropractic vertebral subluxation theory and who limit their practice to the care of neuromusculoskeletal problems of mechanical origin.

National Chiropractic Mutual Insurance Company (NCMIC). The largest chiropractic malpractice insurer in the United States.

Naturopathy. Pseudoscientific approach to health care based on the belief that the basic cause of disease is violation of nature's laws. Its practitioners use dietary measures, fasting, vitamins, herbs, homeopathic remedies, colonic irrigation, and various other modalities, most of which have little or no scientific substantiation.

Nerve root. One of the two nerve bundles emerging from the spinal cord that join to form a segmental spinal nerve.

Neural Organization Technique (N.O.T.). Method purported to "organize" the nervous system and activate helpful reflexes by using applied kinesiology muscle-testing to identify and correct food allergies and dysfunctions claimed to affect the flow of cerebrospinal fluid around the brain.

Nervo-Scope. A handheld, dual-probe thermocouple gadget purported to locate "subluxations" by measuring skin temperature on both sides of the spine.

Neuro Emotional Technique (NET). Method purported to correct disease-causing subluxations that result from negative emotions that "lock in" a "neuro emotional complex (N.E.C)."

Neurocalometer. The heat-detecting instrument originally developed in 1924 for locating subluxated vertebrae.

Neurogenic claudication. Pain and weakness in both legs when standing, which can be relieved by sitting or bending forward. Usually the result of spinal stenosis, a narrowing of the spinal canal (central stenosis) or the openings between the vertebrae (lateral stenosis).

Neurologic deficit. Muscle weakness, loss of sensation, loss of a tendon or muscle reflex, and other symptoms that occur as a result of damage to a spinal nerve.

Nimmo method. Technique that uses digital pressure on trigger points to relax muscles said to be pulling vertebrae out of alignment.

Nonforce techniques. Various reflex techniques and muscle-treatment methods that do not involve forceful manipulation.

NUCCA (National Upper Cervical Association). Organization that promotes upper cervical adjustments to correct the "atlas subluxation complex" ("ASC"). Various questionable upper cervical techniques are used by chiropractors who believe that atlas misalignment is the major subluxation that must be corrected to restore and maintain health.

Orthogonal methods. Upper cervical measurements and techniques that often require use of instruments and machines to correct what are claimed to be minute but all-important subluxations of the atlas.

Osteomalacia. Bone softening caused by a deficiency in vitamin D and inadequate mineralization of new bone. A contraindication for spinal manipulation.

Osteopathic physician (D.O.). Graduate of an osteopathic medical school. The scope of osteopathy is similar to that of medicine except for additional emphasis on the musculoskeletal system. However, some osteopaths advocate the concept of an "osteopathic lesion" (analogous to the chiropractic "subluxation") and claim that manipulation can boost immunity or improve general health.

Osteopenia. A reduction in bone mass to a level just below normal but not enough to contribute to fractures. Early detection of osteopenia by bone density examinations can be helpful in preventing the development of osteoporosis.

Osteoporosis. Brittle or soft bones caused by a variety of contributing factors, such as nutritional deficiency, genetics, low hormone levels, excessive use of cortisone, or prolonged inactivity. Osteoporosis cannot be detected on a plain x-ray examination until at least 30 percent of bone mass has been lost. The appearance of vertebral osteoporosis on x-ray film is a contraindication for spinal manipulation.

Palpate. Touch with the hand, usually as part of a diagnostic examination.

P.A.L. technique (positive anatomical leg length). "New" technique for detecting differences in leg length. Commonly used by chiropractors to do "health screenings" in malls and at health fairs. X-ray examination is then recommended to locate the cause of the deficiency and its effect on the spine, so that correction can be made with spinal and pelvic adjustments. Most structural leg deficiencies with associated compensatory spinal curves and pelvic rotations are not significant and are not correctable.

Parasympathetic nervous system. The set of autonomic nerves emanating from the cranial and sacral areas.

Pettibone method. Upper cervical adjustive technique that utilizes an instrument to adjust the atlas. Orthogonal lines are used to measure the full spine.

Phrenology. Pseudoscience based on the belief that the contours of the skull reflect the person's mental faculties and character.

Pierce-Stillwagon method. Technique similar to Sacro-Occipital Technique which involves contacts and other maneuvers applied to cervical and pelvic areas to produce effects in remote muscles, organs, and joints. A full-spine x-ray examination is considered essential for pelvic analysis. Uses a heat-detecting instrument (Derma Therm-O-Graph) to monitor subluxation correction.

Placebo effect. Favorable response to a treatment that does not result from a pharmacologic effect or other direct physical action.

Portal-of-entry provider. A practitioner whom patients can see without a referral.

Primary-care provider. Health-care professional who provides basic health services, manages routine health-care needs, and is usually the first contact when someone needs care.

Pseudoscience. A theory or method that is falsely represented as scientific. Its proponents typically use scientific terms, distort scientific findings, and/or use anecdotes or testimonials to support their claims.

Quackery. Promotion of health methods that are unsubstantiated and lack a scientifically plausible rationale.

Radiculitis. Inflammation or irritation of a spinal nerve near its origin.

Radiculopathy. General term for nerve-root disorders, most often caused by damage to a spinal nerve, most often as a result of compression caused by disk herniation or spur formation. Pain, loss or decreased sensation of touch, paresthesia (feelings of "pins and needles"), weakness, and decreased reflexes may occur in the distribution of nerves derived from the involved root.

Radiograph. Medical or chiropractic term for an x-ray film.

Radiologist. Specialist trained in the use of radiation for diagnosing and treating disease. Radiologists commonly read and interpret x-ray films for other practitioners.

Referred pain. Pain felt in a part of the body remote from its actual source.

Reflexology. Pseudoscience based on beliefs that each body part is represented on the hands and feet and that pressing on the hands and the soles of the feet can have therapeutic effects in other parts of the body. Some chiropractors use a version of reflexology by pressing into "meridians" in various portions of the body.

Reformist chiropractor. Chiropractor who openly rejects subluxation theories and advocates limiting chiropractic care to musculoskeletal problems of mechanical origin.

Rheumatoid arthritis (RA). An autoimmune disease that erodes joints and supporting tissues. Rheumatoid arthritis is a contraindication for manipulation, especially when the disease affects the atlas and axis at the top of the spine.

Roentgenology. The science of using x-rays for diagnostic purposes.

Sacro-occipital technique. Pseudoscientific diagnostic and treatment method said to involve analysis and correction of sacral and cranial distortions to improve circulation of cerebrospinal fluid. The degree of alleged correction obtained is monitored by checking leg length.

Sacrum. The triangular bone that serves as a base for the spinal column and connects the pelvic bones.

Saddle anesthesia. Loss of sensation in the skin over the perineum (the region between the anus and the genitals). Numbness in this area may be an early indication of disk protrusion into the spinal canal—a contraindication for spinal manipulation.

Scoliosis. Lateral deviation from the normally straight vertical axis of the spine.

Sciatica. Leg pain that originates from lower lumbar and sacral nerves that pass down the back of the thigh into the lower leg and foot.

Self-limiting illness. An illness that resolves with time without treatment. Pseudoscientific practitioners often claim credit for such "cures," as in the case of chiropractic treatment of otitis media.

Short-lever manipulation. A method of spinal manipulation in which contact is made on a vertebral process to move a single vertebra.

SMT. An abbreviation for "spinal manipulative therapy."

Spasm. Involuntary contraction of a muscle or group of muscles.

Spinal "adjustment." A chiropractic term that most chiropractors use to describe whatever method(s) they use to correct spinal problems, whether by hand or with an instrument. Some equate the terms "adjustment" and "manipulation." Others, particularly those who espouse subluxation philosophy, think that the term "adjustment" implies that their method(s) are superior to those of nonchiropractors.

Spinal manipulation. A forceful, high-velocity thrust that stretches a joint beyond its passive range of movement in order to increase its mobility. Manipulation is usually accompanied by an audible pop or click. Because of the speed involved, the patient does not have control and the potential for injury is greater than exists with mobilization.

Spinal stenosis. Narrowing of the spinal canal or vertebral openings that might encroach upon the cauda equina or the spinal nerves, sometimes producing weakness in both legs.

Spondylolisthesis. Slipping forward of one vertebra upon another, often as a result of a congenital defect in the joint structures.

Straight chiropractor. Chiropractors who tend to cling to chiropractic's original doctrine that most health problems are caused by misaligned spinal bones ("vertebral subluxations") and are correctable by manual manipulation of the spine.

Straight leg raising (SLR). A test in which each hip is alternately flexed with the knee extended and the extent to which each leg can be raised is noted. The procedure stretches the sciatic nerve and can reproduce symptoms in the buttock or leg if a spinal nerve-root problem exists.

Stressology. Intricate but nonsensical use of a mathematical analysis to locate stress points in the spinal analysis. Like the gobbledygook of applied kinesiology and some other chiropractic analyses, Stressology is a language that is spoken only by "Stressologists."

Stroke. Sudden loss of brain function caused by blockage or rupture of a blood vessel to the brain. Also called cerebrovascular accident (CVA).

Subluxations. Medical term for partial dislocation of a bone. Chiropractors define "vertebral subluxation" in many ways (see Chapter 4).

Super-straight chiropractors. Chiropractors who believe that their treatment affects "Innate Intelligence." Their sole purpose is said to be locating and correcting vertebral subluxations, rather than diagnosing or treating disease.

Surface EMG scanning (SEMG). An unsubstantiated procedure that measures skin temperature and electrical activity in muscles surrounding the spine. Chiropractors who use it claim that it provides evidence of nerve dysfunction associated with vertebral subluxations. This procedure differs from needle electromyography, a legitimate neurologic test in which needles are inserted into the skin.

Surrogate testing. A senseless method of diagnosing problems by testing the muscle strength of a third person who is touching the patient. Some chiropractors use this method to diagnose allergies, deficiencies, and other alleged problems in infants and small children.

Sweat method. Atlas orthogonal technique in which the atlas is adjusted using a special table and a solenoid stylus placed against the side of the neck just behind and below the ear.

Sympathetic nervous system. The set of autonomic nerves emanating from the thoracic and lumbar areas of the spine.

"Ten danger signals." A list of common symptoms allegedly caused by pinched nerves or misaligned vertebra.

Therapeutic touch. An invalid but widely used nursing practice whose practitioners claim to heal or improve many medical problems by manual manipulation of a "human energy field" perceptible above the patient's skin.

Thermography. A diagnostic procedure that images heat from body surfaces. Commonly used by chiropractors but has not been found to be effective in locating pinched nerves or subluxated vertebrae.

Thompson terminal point technique. A chiropractic adjustment performed on a table in which the supporting cushions drop an inch or two when a thrust is applied to the spine. Practitioners locate "subluxations" by checking leg lengths with the legs straight, the knees bent, or the head turned to either side.

Thoracic outlet syndrome. Collective title for several vascular or neurologic conditions in which blood vessels or nerve fibers (brachial plexus) are known or assumed to be compromised at any point between the base of the neck and the armpit.

Thoracic vertebrae. There are twelve vertebrae in the thoracic or upper-back portion of the spine.

Toftness method. Method in which a handheld "Toftness Radiation Detector" is used to locate subluxated vertebrae and pinched nerves so that they can then be corrected with spinal adjustments. Although the FDA has banned the device, a few chiropractors still use it.

Toggle recoil technique. Manipulation performed with a sudden shallow thrust (toggle) followed by quick withdrawal (recoil) of the chiropractor's hands while the patient is relaxed.

Total body modification (T.B.M.). Method that involves locating stressed organs or body areas so that "tried and tested reflex points and muscle testing" can be used to stimulate specific areas of the spine. This supposedly restores balance to the nervous system by stimulating nerve cells in the brain, which enables the brain to regain control of the body and guide it back to health.

Traction (of the spine). Stretching of the spine by hand or with equipment, to relieve compression on joints or disks.

Transverse process. Bony protrusion on either side of the arch of a vertebra, which functions as a lever for attached muscles.

True believer. Someone who is deeply, sometimes fanatically, devoted to a cause, organization, or person.

Upper cervical specific. Technique that uses a number of specific chiropractic adjustments designed to correct atlas and upper cervical subluxations.

Vertebra. Bony segment of the spine that encircles and helps protect the spinal cord and nerves. The plural of vertebra is vertebrae.

Vertebral artery. Arteries, one on each side, that thread through holes in the six upper cervical vertebrae. Sudden rotation during neck manipulation can injure them and interrupt blood flow to the lower part of the brain, causing a stroke.

Vertebral subluxation complex. A "modern" chiropractic term for the chiropractic subluxation.

Viscera. The soft internal organs of the body, especially those contained within the abdominal and thoracic cavities.

Vitalism. The concept that the functions of an organism are due to a "vital principle" or "life force" distinct from the physical forces explainable by the laws of physics and chemistry. Chiropractors refer to that force as "Innate Intelligence."

World Chiropractic Alliance (WCA). An organization of chiropractors, students, and laypersons that promotes super-straight chiropractic.

"Yet disease." A technique for selling chiropractic care by asking people whether they have experienced various symptoms "yet."

Appendix E

References

1. ACA policies on public health and related matters. Journal of the American Chiropractic Association 34(3):33–52, 1997.
2. Aker PD, Martel J. Maintenance care. Topics in Clinical Chiropractic 3(4):32–35, 1996.
3. Alliance for Chiropractic Progress. $1.8 million and counting: ACA/ICA Alliance for Chiropractic Progress (advertisement). The American Chiropractor 20(6):24–30, 1998.
4. Alliance for Chiropractic Progress. Whole body healing (advertisement). Prevention 50(4):25, 1998.
5. AMA Dept. of Investigation. Admission to schools of chiropractic. JAMA 190(8):153–154, 1963.
6. AMA Dept. of Investigation. Educational background of chiropractic school faculties. JAMA 197(12):169–175, 1966.
7. American Academy of Neurology, Therapeutics and Technology Assessment Subcommittee. Assessment: Thermography in neurologic practice. Neurology 40:523–525, 1990.
8. American Chiropractic Association. 1993 Public Relations Guide. October Is Spinal Health Month. ACA Journal of Chiropractic 30(8):SP2–SP3, 1993.
9. American Chiropractic Association. *Chiropractic: State of the Art, 1994–1995.* Arlington, VA: American Chiropractic Association, 1994.
10. American College of Radiology. Ultrasound: Not effective in diagnosing spinal injuries. ACR Bulletin 2-96, Feb. 1996.
11. An integrative medicine primer (booklet). Boston: Integrative Medicine Communications, 1998, p. 3.
12. Armstrong D, Armstrong E. *The Great American Medicine Show.* New York, NY: Prentice Hall, 1991, pp. 139–137.

13. Association of Chiropractic Colleges. A position paper on chiropractic. JMPT 19:634–637, 1996.
14. Baker R. Letters to the Editor. Chiropractic Technique 4(4):155, 1992.
15. Balon J et al. A comparison of active and simulated chiropractic manipulation as adjunctive treatment for childhood asthma. New England Journal of Medicine 339:1013–1020, 1998.
16. Barge F. Final thoughts: Possibly true? Today's Chiropractic 22(4):105, 1993.
17. Barrett S. Applied kinesiology: Muscle-testing for "allergies" and "nutrient deficiencies," Quackwatch Web site, 1998.
18. Barrett S. Commercial hair analysis: Science or scam? JAMA 254:1041–1045, 1985.
19. Barrett S. Dubious aspects of osteopathy. Quackwatch Web site, 1998.
20. Barrett S. "Electrodiagnostic" devices. Quackwatch Web site, 1998.
21. Barrett S. The herbal minefield. Quackwatch Web site, 1998.
22. Barrett S. The spine salesmen. In Barrett S, editor. *The New Health Robbers: How to Save Your Money and Your Life*. Philadelphia PA: George F. Stickley Co., 1980.
23. Barrett S et al. *Consumer Health: A Guide to Intelligent Decisions*, 6th Edition. Madison, WI: Brown & Benchmark, 1997.
24. Barrett S, Herbert V. *The Vitamin Pushers: How the "Health Food" Industry Is Selling America a Bill of Goods*. Amherst, NY: Prometheus Books, 1994.
25. Best H, Taylor N. *The Physiological Basis of Medical Practice*, 5th Edition. Baltimore, MD: Williams & Wilkins, 1950, p. 286.
26. Bigos SJ. AHCPR low back guidelines and chiropractic care. Dynamic Chiropractic 13(10):41, 1995.
27. Bigos SJ et al. *Acute Low Back Pain Problems in Adults*. Clinical Practice Guideline No. 14. AHCPR Publication No. 95-0642. Rockville, MD: Agency for Health Care Policy & Research, 1994.
28. Blue Pages. In *National Directory of Chiropractic*, 7th Edition 1996–1997. Olathe, KS: One Directory of Chiropractic, Inc., 1996.
29. Botnick AJ. Some notes on Life College's assembly and its money hum. Chirobase Web site, 1999.
30. Bove G, Nilsson N. Spinal manipulation in the treatment of episodic tension-type headache. JAMA 280:1576–1579, 1998.
31. Brennan P et al. Enhanced neutrophil respiratory burst induced by spinal manipulation: Potential role of substance P. JMPT 14:399–408, 1991.
32. Burney L. *Report to the Secretary of Health, Education, and Welfare on the 1958 Poliomyelitis Season*. Washington, DC: U.S. Public Health Service, 1958.
33. Callender A, Plaugher G, Anrig CA. Introduction to chiropractic pediatrics. In Anrig CA, Plaugher G (editors). *Pediatric Chiropractic*. Baltimore: Williams & Wilkins, 1998.
34. Casura LG. Interview with Scott Walker, D.C., founder of neuroemotional technique (NET), and Steve Shaffer, an NET practitioner. Townsend Letter for Doctors & Patients, July 1998, pp. 128–134.

35. Cherkin DC et al. A comparison of physical therapy, chiropractic manipulation, and provision of an educational booklet for the treatment of patients with low back pain. New England Journal of Medicine 339:1021–1029, 1998.

36. Cherkin D et al. *Chiropractic in the United States: Training, Practice, and Research.* Rockville, MD: Agency for Health Care Policy and Research, 1997. U.S. Department of Commerce publication PB9111693.

37. Chiropractors. Consumer Reports 59:383–390, 1994.

38. Christenson MG, Morgan DRD. *Job Analysis of Chiropractic: A Report, Survey Analysis, and Summary of the Practice of Chiropractic within the United States.* Greeley, CO: National Board of Chiropractic Examiners, 1993.

39. Cianculli AE. Chiropractic: A primary care gatekeeper. Arlington, VA: American Chiropractic Association Political Action Committee, 1992.

40. Cockburn DM. A study of the validity of iris diagnosis. Australian Journal of Optometry 64:154–157, 1981.

41. Cohen MR. When you visit a Chinese medicine practitioner. Downloaded from http://acupuncture.com/Diagnosis/firsttreat.htm, Dec. 29, 1998.

42. Cohen WJ. *Independent Practitioners Under Medicare: A Report to Congress.* Washington, DC: U.S. Department of Health, Education, and Welfare, 1968.

43. Colley F, Haas M. Attitudes on immunization: A survey of American chiropractors. JMPT 17:584–590, 1994.

44. Committee on the Future of Primary Care. *Primary Care: America's Health in a New Era.* Washington, DC: National Academy Press, 1994.

45. Conragan, N. Nicole Conragan Clinic Web site (http://www.businessquest.com/chiropractor), downloaded Jan. 27, 1999.

46. Contact Reflex Analysis and Designed Clinical Nutrition hands-on training, March 14–15, 1998. Flyer, Dallas TX: Parker College of Chiropractic, 1998.

47. Cooke P. The Crescent City cure. Hippocrates 2(6):61–70, 1988.

48. Cooper R, Staflet S. Trends in the education and practice of alternative medicine clinicians. Health Affairs 15:226–252, 1996.

49. Coulter I et al. *The Appropriateness of Manipulation and Mobilization of the Cervical Spine.* Santa Monica, CA: RAND, 1996, pp. 18–43.

50. Council on Chiropractic Education. *Standards for Chiropractic Programs and Institutions.* Scottsdale, AZ: Council on Chiropractic Education, 1995.

51. Crelin ES. A scientific test of the chiropractic theory. American Scientist 61:574–580, 1973.

52. Crelin ES. Chiropractic. In Stalker D, Glymour C (editors). *Examining Holistic Medicine.* Amherst, NY: Prometheus Books, 1989.

53. Cyriax J. *Textbook of Orthopedic Medicine.* London: Cassell, 1955.

54. DeJarnette M. *Sacro Occipital Technic of Chiropractic.* Nebraska City, NE, 1952.

55. Doxey TT, Phillips RB. Comparison of entrance requirements for health care professions. JMPT 20:86–91, 1997.

56. Ernst E, Eckhart GH, editors. *Homeopathy: A Critical Appraisal.* Oxford, England: Butterworth-Heinemann, 1998.

57. Fact sheet on chiropractic. Lombard, IL: National College of Chiropractic, 1998.
58. Ferguson A, Weise G. How many chiropractic schools? An analysis of institutions that offered the D.C. degree. Chiropractic History 8(1):27–36, 1988.
59. Fernandez PG. What you have to do differently today to increase your practice. The American Chiropractor 20(3):30–31, 1998.
60. Fishbein M. *The Medical Follies.* New York: Boni and Liveright, 1925, p. 89.
61. Fisher A. *Treatment by Manipulation.* London, England: H.K. Lewis & Company, Ltd., 1948, pp. 11–14, 265.
62. FTC questions Koren's claims. Is Koren Publications just the beginning? Dynamic Chiropractic, Sept. 21, 1998, pp. 1,17,42,49.
63. Frame F. Has the test tube fight against polio failed? Journal of the National Chiropractic Association, March 1959.
64. Fuhr AW. *Activator Methods Chiropractic Technique.* St. Louis: Mosby, 1997, p. 92.
65. Getzendanner S. Memorandum opinion and order in *Wilk et al v AMA et al,* No. 76 C 3777, US District Court for the Northern District of Illinois, Eastern Division, August 27, 1987.
66. Gevitz N. *The D.O.'s: Osteopathic Medicine in America.* Baltimore: The Johns Hopkins University Press, 1982.
67. Gibbons RW. The Rise of the chiropractic educational establishment, 1897–1980. In Lints-Dzaman F (editorial director). *Who's Who in Chiropractic International,* 2nd Edition. Littleton, CO: Who's Who in Chiropractic International Publishing Co., 1980, pp. 339–352.
68. Gray P. Tips for training your receptionist. In *477 Practice Building & Office Procedure Ideas: The Best of Share, Volume I.* Ft. Worth, TX: Parker Chiropractic Research Foundation, 1977.
69. Gregg RJ. Endorsement in ad from Precision Technology, Inc. Today's Chiropractic 21(3):51, 1992.
70. Haggard H. *Devils, Drugs, and Doctors.* New York, NY: Blue Ribbon Books, 1929, p. 39.
71. Haldeman S, Chapman-Smith D, Peterson D. *Guidelines for Chiropractic Quality Assurance and Practice Parameters: Proceedings of the Mercy Center Consensus Conference.* Gaithersburg, MD: Aspen Publishers, 1993, pp. 107–108.
72. Hambidge KM. Hair analyses: Worthless for vitamins, limited for minerals. American Journal of Clinical Nutrition 36:943–949, 1983.
73. Harmon JC. Incorporating holistic medicine into equine practice. In *Alternative and Complementary Veterinary Medicine: Principles and Practices.* St. Louis: Mosby, 1998, pp. 631–647.
74. Harrison JD. Diagnosis: Pros, cons and limitations. In Harrison JD. *Chiropractic Practice Liability: A Guide to Successful Risk Management.* Arlington, VA: International Chiropractors Association, 1990, pp. 112–116.
75. Hawk C, Dusio M. A survey of 492 U.S. chiropractors on primary care and prevention-related issues. JMPT 18:57–64, 1995.

76. Henderson D et al. *Clinical Guidelines for Chiropractic Practice in Canada.* Toronto: Canadian Chiropractic Association, 1994.
77. Hippocrates. *Great Books of the Western World, Volume 10, Hippocrates, Galen.* Chicago: Encyclopædia Britannica, 1952, pp. 106–114.
78. Ho M. Acupuncture and chiropractic: Is there a link? Journal of the American Chiropractic Association 35(3):13–14, 1998.
79. Homewood AE. *The Neurodynamics of the Vertebral Subluxation,* 3d Edition. St. Petersburg, FL: Valkyrie Press, 1977.
80. Homola S. *Bonesetting, Chiropractic, and Cultism.* Panama City, FL: Critique Books, 1963.
81. Homola S. Chiropractic and your back. Muscular Development 20(3):14–56, 1983.
82. Homola S. Chiropractic as a neuromusculoskeletal specialty. Chiropractic Technique 7(4):147–148, 1995.
83. Homola S. Finding a good chiropractor. Archives of Family Medicine 7:20–23, 1998.
84. Homola S. Seeking a common denominator in the use of spinal manipulation. Chiropractic Technique 4(2):61–63, 1992.
85. Homola S. Sense and nonsense in chiropractic care of the back. Scholastic Coach and Athletic Director 64(8):32–35, 1995.
86. Homola S. Thirty years after Bonesetting, Chiropractic, and Cultism: Confessions of a chiropractic heretic. Chiropractic History 15(2):15–18, 1995.
87. How DCs in the USA practice. Dynamic Chiropractic 6(17):3, 1988.
88. Hurwitz E et al. Use of chiropractic services from 1985 through 1991 in the United States and Canada. American Journal of Public Health 88:771–776, 1998.
89. Hyde T. Letter to Samuel Homola, May 13, 1995.
90. ICAK-U.S.A. Executive Board. Letter to Stephen Barrett, M.D., Nov. 11, 1998. Quackwatch Web site, 1998.
91. International Conference on Chiropractic and Pediatrics. Presented by International Chiropractic Association, cosponsored by Palmer College of Chiropractic. Sept. 19–21, 1997.
92. Ivanchuk J. Letters to the Editor. Chiropractic Technique 4(4):156, 1992.
93. Janse J, Houser R, Wells B. *Chiropractic Principles and Technic,* 2d Edition. Chicago, IL: National College of Chiropractic, 1947: 15–32.
94. Jansen RD, Meeker W, Rosner A. American chiropractors' research priorities. Journal of the Neuromusculoskeletal System 5(4):144–149, 1997.
95. Jarvis WT, editor. Homeopathy: A position statement by the National Council Against Health Fraud. Skeptic 3(1):50–57, 1994.
96. Jensen B. *Iridology Simplified.* Escondido, CA: Iridologists International, 1980.
97. Johnson SM et al. Variables influencing the use of osteopathic manipulative treatment in family practice. Journal of the American Osteopathic Association 97:80–87, 1997.
98. Kale MU. "Houston Control": The master control system of the human body (http://www.kale.com/kale2.html); and Kale Network . . . Dr. Kale (http://www.kale.com/kale4.html). Downloaded Dec. 12, 1998.

99. Kaufman Chiropractic, Madison, Wisconsin. Downloaded Jan 24, 1999. (States that referral from a veterinarian is required.)

100. Keating J. Chiropractic professional associations. In *Chiropractic: An Illustrated History*. St. Louis: Mosby, 1995, pp. 421–443.

101. Keating J. Chiropractic: science and antiscience and pseudoscience side by side. Skeptical Inquirer 21(4):37–43, 1997.

102. Keating JC Jr. Slow progress. Dynamic Chiropractic 11(23):44, 1993.

103. Keating J. *Toward a Philosophy of the Science of Chiropractic*. Stockton, CA: Stockton Foundation for Chiropractic Research, 1992, pp. 76–84.

104. Kent C, Gentempo P Jr. Paraspinal surface EMG: Its role in chiropractic practice. Today's Chiropractic 22(3):14–16, 66, 1993.

105. King FJ Jr. The marriage of chiropractic and homeopathy. Interview. The American Chiropractor 13(2):7–11, 1991.

106. King FJ Jr. Using homeopathy to enhance a high volume practice. King Bio Pharmaceuticals Web site, downloaded Dec. 24, 1998.

107. Klemis DE. *The New Patient Orientation*. Lecture and slides. Beverly, MA: Chiropractic Educational Systems, 1993.

108. Knipschild P. Looking for gall bladder disease in the patient's iris. British Medical Journal 297:1578–1581, 1988.

109. Koes BW et al. Spinal manipulation for low back pain: An updated systematic review of randomized clinical trials. Spine 21:2860–2873, 1996.

110. Koren T. Chiropractic: Bringing out the best in you. Philadelphia: Koren Publications, 1995.

111. Koren T. How to create million-dollar-plus practices. Philadelphia: Koren Publications, undated.

112. Koren T. How to get 5 to 10 new patients a week without leaving your office. Philadelphia: Koren Publications, 1996.

113. Koren T. Is vaccination a chiropractic issue? Today's Chiropractic 16(6):86–87, 1997.

114. Lamm LC, Wegner E, Collord D. Chiropractic scope of practice: What the law allows—update 1993. JMPT 18:16–20, 1995.

115. Leach RA. *The Chiropractic Theories: A Synopsis of Scientific Research*. Baltimore: Williams & Wilkins, 1986.

116. *Life College Bulletin, 1996–1997*. Marietta, GA: Life University, 1996, p. 58.

117. Logan H. *Textbook of Logan Basic Methods*. St. Louis: Logan Basic College of Chiropractic, 1950.

118. Loomis H. Combining nutrition and chiropractic. The American Chiropractor 20(6):24–25,33, 1998.

119. *Los Angeles College of Chiropractic Academic Catalogue*. Whittier, CA, 1997–1999, p. 17.

120. Magner G. *Chiropractic: The Victim's Perspective*. Amherst, NY: Prometheus Books, 1995.

121. Martin EZ. The Micro-Dynameter. Journal of Micro-Dynameter Research (8-page brochure). Chicago, Ellis Research Laboratories, 1954.

122. Martin SC. Chiropractic and American science: 1895–1990. Isis 85:207–227, 1994.

123. Mennell J. *The Science and Art of Joint Manipulation: The Spinal Column.* New York, NY: The Blakiston Company, 1952, pp. 2–4.

124. Menninger B. Student policies questioned in school verdict. Kansas City Business Journal, July 12–18, 1996, pp. 1,42.

125. Meyerhoff E. Book review: Bonesetting, Chiropractic, and Cultism. Library Journal 89:643, 1964.

126. Moran WC et al. *Inspection of Chiropractic Services Under Medicare.* Chicago: OIG Office of Analysis & Inspections, 1986.

127. Nasel D, Szlazak M. Somatic dysfunction and the phenomenon of visceral disease simulation: a probable explanation for the apparent effectiveness of somatic therapy in patients presumed to be suffering from true visceral disease. JMPT 18(6):379–397, 1995.

128. Nelson C. Letter to the Editor. Chiropractic Technique 4:158, 1992.

129. Nelson C. Scope of practice. JMPT 16:488–497, 1993.

130. Nelson C. The subluxation question. Journal of Chiropractic Humanitics 7:46–55, 1997.

131. Nelson C. Why chiropractors should embrace immunization. Journal of the American Chiropractic Association 30(5):79–85, 1993.

132. Nikitow D. Patient education. ICA International Review of Chiropractic 53(6):51–55, 1997.

133. Palmer BJ. Palmer tells benefits of advertising. Fountain Head News. November 1, 1919.

134. Palmer BJ. *Shall Chiropractic Survive?* 1st Edition. Davenport, IA: Palmer School of Chiropractic, 1958.

135. Palmer BJ. *Shall Chiropractic Survive?* 2d Edition. Davenport, IA: Palmer School of Chiropractic, 1959.

136. Palmer BJ. *The Science of Chiropractic: Its Principles & Adjustments.* Davenport, IA: The Palmer School of Chiropractic, 1906.

137. Palmer DD. *The Chiropractor's Adjuster: A Text-Book of the Science, Art and Philosophy of Chiropractic.* Portland, OR: Portland Printing House Company, 1910.

138. Palmer DD. The Magnetic Cure, Jan. 1896, Number 15. Cited in Keating JC Jr. *Toward a Philosophy of the Science of Chiropractic.* Stockton, CA: Stockton Foundation for Chiropractic Research, 1992.

139. *Palmer College of Chiropractic Catalog.* Davenport, IA, 1997–1998, pp. 6–8, 21.

140. Parker JW. *Textbook of Office Procedure and Practice Building for the Chiropractic Profession,* 4th Edition. Ft. Worth, TX: Parker Chiropractic Research Foundation, Inc., 1975.

141. Peet J. Chiropractic analysis of the newborn infant. Journal of Clinical Chiropractic 8(3):26–27, 1998.

142. Peterson D, Weise G. *Chiropractic: An Illustrated History.* St. Louis: Mosby-Year Book, 1995.

143. Pierce WV. Results. Dravosberg, PA: CHIRP, 1981.
144. Plasker E. Traumatic birth syndrome and the need for infant spinal care. Today's Chiropractic 27(1):24–33, 1998.
145. Pottenger F. *Symptoms of Visceral Disease*, 7th Edition. St. Louis, MO: C.V. Mosby Company, 1953, p. 82.
146. *Practice Guidelines for Straight Chiropractic*. Chandler, AZ: World Chiropractic Alliance, 1993, p. 30.
147. Pruitt H. Letter to Samuel Homola, May 17, 1965.
148. Quigley WH. Chiropractic's monocausal theory of disease. ACA Journal of Chiropractic 18(6):52–60, 1981.
149. Readers respond to Dr. Homola. The Chiropractic Journal 9(11):8–9, 1995.
150. Redding D. Letter to Samuel Homola, July 1, 1991.
151. Referrals to the chiropractic lifestyle (pamphlet). Colorado Springs, CO: Back Talk Systems, 1995.
152. Rome PL. Usage of chiropractic terminology in the literature: 296 ways to say "subluxation": complex issues of the vertebral subluxation. Chiropractic Technique 8:49–60, 1996.
153. Rondberg T. *Chiropractic First*. Chandler, AZ: The Chiropractic Journal, 1996, pp. 3, 88.
154. Roney J. Stanford Research Institute. Personal correspondence, November 11, 1965.
155. Rosner AL. *The Role of Subluxation in Chiropractic*. Des Moines, IA: Foundation for Chiropractic Research, 1997.
156. Rosner AL. What subluxation means to you (pamphlet). Des Moines, IA: Foundation for Chiropractic Research, 1997.
157. Sampson W et al. Acupuncture: The position paper of the National Council Against Health Fraud. Clinical Journal of Pain 7:162–166, 1991.
158. Savage T. What is N.O.T.? Neural organization Technique and what it can do for me. N.O.T. Homepage (http://www.st.net.au/~welbeing/not.htm). Downloaded Jan. 21, 1999.
159. Schafer RC. *Basic Chiropractic Procedural Manual, Volume 1*. Arlington, VA: American Chiropractic Association, 1973.
160. Schafer RC. *Developing a Chiropractic Practice: An Introduction to Tactical Chiropractic Economics*. Arlington, VA: American Chiropractic Association, 1984.
161. Seater S. Letter to the Editor. Chiropractic Technique 8(2):93–94, 1996.
162. Shekelle PG. RAND misquoted. Journal of the American Chiropractic Association 30(7):59–63, 1993.
163. Shekelle PG. What role for chiropractic in health care? New England Journal of Medicine 339:1074–1075, 1998.
164. Shekelle PG et al. Congruence between decisions to initiate chiropractic spinal manipulation for low back pain and appropriate criteria in North America. Annals of Internal Medicine 129:9–17, 1998.

165. Shekelle PG et al. *The Appropriateness of Spinal Manipulation for Low-Back Pain. Part I. Project Overview and Literature Review. Part II. Indications and Ratings by a Multidisciplinary Expert Panel. Part III. Indications and Ratings by an All-Chiropractic Expert Panel.* Santa Monica, CA: RAND Corporation, 1991–1992.

166. Shenker GR. *An Analytical System of Clinical Nutrition.* Mifflintown, PA: NUTRI-SPEC, 1989.

167. Sherman College of Straight Chiropractic. *The Philosophy, Science, & Art of Straight Chiropractic.* Bulletin, 1997–1998, pp. 9–10.

168. Sherr JY. *The Dynamics and Methodology of Provings.* West Malvern, England: Dynamis Books, 1994.

169. Simon A et al. An evaluation of iridology. JAMA 242:1385–1387, 1979.

170. Singer D. Pamphlets: (a) Relief care (1993); (b) Corrective care (1993); (c) Maintenance care (1993); and (d) Children and chiropractic (1990). Clearwater, FL: Expand Chiropractic Products.

171. Smith J. Killer subluxations. The American Chiropractor 19(4):23–32, 1997.

172. Smith M. Letter to "Dear Colleague." April, 1995.

173. Smith RL. *At Your Own Risk: The Case against Chiropractic.* New York: Pocket Books, 1969.

174. Smith T. Chiropractors seeking to expand practices take aim at children. The Wall Street Journal, March 18, 1993, pp. A1, A4.

175. Social Security Amendments of 1972 (Public Law 92-603), Oct. 30, 1972, pp. 123–134.

176. Sollmann AH, Blaurock-Busch E. Manipulative therapy of the spine: The development of 'manual medicine' in Germany and Europe. Chiropractic History 1(1):37–41, 1981.

177. Sottile, RT. Mandatory Immunization and You? A Must for All Parents to Read! Marietta, GA: Life Foundation, circa 1976.

178. Speer T. Letter to the Editor. Muscular Development 20(5):6, 1983.

179. Spock B. Easing the pain of ear infection. Parenting, Feb. 1998, pp. 82–85.

180. Sportelli L. *Introduction to Chiropractic: A Natural Method of Healthcare*, 9th Edition. Palmerton, PA: Practice Makers Products, Inc., 1988, pp. 6,7,10,22.

181. Sportelli L. 20/20 vision or blindness? ACA Journal of Chiropractic 31(3):58–59, 68–69, 1994.

182. Stanford Research Institute. *Chiropractic in California.* Los Angeles, CA: The Haynes Foundation, 1960, p. 9.

183. Still AT. *Autobiography—with a history of the discovery and development of the science of osteopathy.* Reprinted, New York, 1972, Arno Press and the New York Times.

184. Stillwagon G, Stillwagon BS. Objective proof: Thermography documents chiropractic efficacy. Today's Chiropractic 23(3):52–56, 1994.

185. Strauss, JB. *Refined by Fire: The Evolution of Straight Chiropractic.* Levittown, PA: Foundation for the Advancement of Chiropractic Education, 1994.

186. Terrett A. *Vertebrobasilar Stroke Following Manipulation.* West Des Moines, IA: National Chiropractic Mutual Insurance Company, 1996.
187. Thank you for being a dedicated and loyal patient of chiropractic care. A recent study by the federal government proves you were correct in selecting spinal manipulation because of its safe and effective benefits (pamphlet). Arlington, VA: American Chiropractic Association, 1995.
188. Tiscareno L, Amalu W. HIO: Old problems, new solutions. Today's Chiropractic 26(6):24–34, 1997.
189. Tosolt A. Chiropractic News Publishing Company. Personal correspondence, Oct. 23, 1984.
190. Versendaal D, Ulan F. Contact reflex analysis and applied clinical nutrition: An effective analytical tool for the alternative health care professional. The American Chiropractor 20(2):18–20, 32, 1998.
191. Wardwell W. *Chiropractic: History and Evolution of a New Profession.* St. Louis, MO: Mosby-Year Book, 1992, pp. 19, 287.
192. Watkins CO. *The Basic Principles of Chiropractic Government.* Self-published, 1944. Reproduced in Keating JC Jr. *Toward a Philosophy of the Science of Chiropractic.* Stockton, CA: Stockton Foundation for Chiropractic Research, 1992.
193. WCA members vote on 'silent killer' terminology. The Chiropractic Journal 6(8):12, 1992.
194. Weiant CW. *Medicine and Chiropractic.* New York, NY: Self-published, 1958, pp. 82–83, 61.
195. Wells D. Think Acu-practic: Acupuncture benefits for chiropractic. Journal of the American Chiropractic Association 35(3):10–13, 1998.
196. What we teach. The Chiropractic Journal 8(1):34–36, 1993.
197. White A. *Your Aching Back: A Doctor's Guide to Relief.* New York, NY: Fireside Books, 1990, p. 54.
198. Williams DG. *The Unauthorized Guide to Nutritional Products & Their Uses.* Ingram, TX: Mountain Home Publishing Co., 1989.
199. Williams SE. *Dynamic Essentials Seminars Procedures Manual.* Marietta, GA: DE International, undated, circa 1991, purchased in 1999.
200. Williams SE. Learning a lesson from the snake oil salesman. Today's Chiropractic 27(1):6–10, 1998.
201. Willoughby S. Chiropractic care. In Schoen AM, Wynn SG. *Alternative and Complementary Veterinary Medicine: Principles and Practices.* St. Louis: Mosby, 1998, pp. 185–200.
202. Winterstein J. Letter to the Editor. Chiropractic Technique 4:157, 1992.
203. Winterstein J. NCC Outreach 14(1):1, 1998.
204. Woodwell DA. National Ambulatory Medical Care Survey: 1996 Summary. National Center for Health Statistics: Advance Data Number 295, Dec. 17, 1997.
205. Zygmont Chiropractic Center Web site (http://www.eden.com/~zyg), downloaded Dec. 20, 1998.

Index

259